SUPPLEMENTS FOR MENTAL HEALTH

FOCUS ON VITAMIN D_3 AND OMEGA 3

SHARMILLA KANAGASUNDRAM

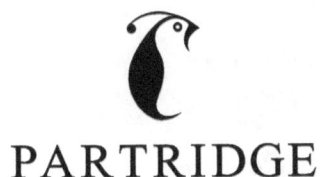

PARTRIDGE

Copyright © 2020 by Sharmilla Kanagasundram.

ISBN:	Softcover	978-1-5437-5907-5
	eBook	978-1-5437-5906-8

All rights reserved. No part of this book may be used or reproduced by any means, graphic, electronic, or mechanical, including photocopying, recording, taping or by any information storage retrieval system without the written permission of the author except in the case of brief quotations embodied in critical articles and reviews.

Because of the dynamic nature of the Internet, any web addresses or links contained in this book may have changed since publication and may no longer be valid. The views expressed in this work are solely those of the author and do not necessarily reflect the views of the publisher, and the publisher hereby disclaims any responsibility for them.

Print information available on the last page.

To order additional copies of this book, contact
Toll Free +65 3165 7531 (Singapore)
Toll Free +60 3 3099 4412 (Malaysia)
orders.singapore@partridgepublishing.com

www.partridgepublishing.com/singapore

AUTHORS

1) **DATIN DR SHARMILLA KANAGASUNDRAM MBBS (MANIPAL), MPM (UM)** Associate Professor, Department of Psychological Medicine, University Malaya.

2) **DR NAVIN NAIR MBBS (MANIPAL), MRCPsych (UK)**

3) **DR NORMINA BINTI AHMAD BUSTAMI MD (UNIMAS), MHSc (UKM)** Assistant Professor, Faculty of Medicine and Health Sciences, UCSI University.

PROLOGUE

Supplements have generally been given little attention by medical practitioners who tend to focus on treating diseased states. While it is important to excel in the treatment of disease it is also prudent to pay attention to the nutritional needs of the body. With careful use of supplementation we might be able to improve immunity, induce a less inflammatory status of the body as well as enlist the help of antioxidants in maintaining a healthy milleu within the body. There are many vitamins and minerals in food that promote and maintain good health. In this book the authors have focused on how some supplements may be useful in certain psychiatric disorders. The supplements elaborated on are vitamin D_3 as well as omega 3. It is not quite understood how nutritional deficiencies interact with genetics, interfere in the serotonin pathway, play an important role in brain development, social cognition, decision-making, and how the gene-environment interactions initiate mental disorders.

The mental disorders that have been addressed in this book are depressive disorders, bipolar disorders and schizophrenia. Cognitive dysfunction can occur in depressive disorders, bipolar disorders, schizophrenia as well as the different types of dementia. Depressive disorders, bipolar disorders and schizophrenia are broad categories as each condition is actually heterogenous in nature as evidenced by multiple genes implicated in each condition that in turn give a very different clinical picture for patients of each disorder. For example: In a group of 100 schizophrenic patients, their symptoms would be variable from one patient to another. Schizophrenia and bipolar patients have various degrees of cognitive dysfunction enabling some to be able to find a job and others to not. Depression generally has a better outcome with most patients being able to function. This being said, cognitive dysfunction is also present albeit to a milder degree in depressive disorders.

Traditional methods of depression treatment using pharmacotherapy such as antidepressants have limitations to their effectiveness. Biological, psychological and environmental causes of depressive disorders are known, but exact pathophysiology of depression is not as yet fully understood. Multiple mechanisms play a role in the pathophysiology of depression, one of which has been postulated to be vitamin D_3 deficiency.

Deficiency or borderline levels of vitamin D_3 is common amongst the general population and may occur even in one billion people globally. Epidemiological studies show that vitamin D_3 or its metabolites do not reach optimal levels in many adults. Even lower than the optimal level might lead to clinical symptoms and risk the individual getting depressed. Patients suffering from depressive disorders have deficiency of vitamin D_3 more frequently than the non- depressed population. Literature on the possible impact of vitamin D_3 deficiency on the prevalence of depression and antidepressant effect of the supplementation is discussed in this book along with effects of omega 3 on the above mentioned psychiatric disorders.

ACKNOWLEDGEMENT

This book is made possible as I was granted sabbatical leave by the University of Malaya between December 2019 and September 2020.

CONTENTS

PROLOGUE..VII
ACKNOWLEDGEMENT.. IX

CHAPTER 1　INTRODUCTION TO VITAMIN D_3................1
Associate Professor Datin Dr Sharmilla Kanagasundram

CHAPTER 2　VITAMIN D_3 AND COGNITION....................5
Associate Professor Datin Dr Sharmilla Kanagasundram

CHAPTER 3　VITAMIN D_3 AND DEPRESSION....................7
Associate Professor Datin Dr Sharmilla Kanagasundram

CHAPTER 4　VITAMIN D_3 AND BIPOLAR DISORDERS...13
Associate Professor Datin Dr Sharmilla Kanagasundram

CHAPTER 5　VITAMIN D_3 AND SCHIZOPHRENIA..........16
Associate Professor Datin Dr Sharmilla Kanagasundram

CHAPTER 6　INTRODUCTION TO OMEGA 3....................24
Associate Professor Datin Dr Sharmilla Kanagasundram

CHAPTER 7　OMEGA 3 AND COGNITION........................30
Associate Professor Datin Dr Sharmilla Kanagasundram

**CHAPTER 8　OMEGA -3 FATTY ACIDS AND
　　　　　　　DEPRESSIVE DISORDERS**........................33
Associate Professor Datin Dr Sharmilla Kanagasundram

CHAPTER 9　OMEGA 3 AND BIPOLAR DISORDER..........40
Associate Professor Datin Dr Sharmilla Kanagasundram

CHAPTER 10 OMEGA 3 AND SCHIZOPHRENIA 44
Associate Professor Datin Dr Sharmilla Kanagasundram

CHAPTER 11 INTRODUCTION TO MAGNESIUM 49
Associate Professor Datin Dr Sharmilla Kanagasundram

CHAPTER 12 INTRODUCTION TO FOLATE 54
Associate Professor Datin Dr Sharmilla Kanagasundram

CHAPTER 13 INTRODUCTION TO ZINC 62
Associate Professor Datin Dr Sharmilla Kanagasundram

CHAPTER 14 COGNITION AS A FUNCTION OF
             THE BRAIN 72
Associate Professor Datin Dr Sharmilla Kanagasundram

CHAPTER 15 OVERVIEW OF MAJOR DEPRESSIVE
             DISORDER 79
Dr Navin Nair Narayanan

CHAPTER 16 OVERVIEW OF BIPOLAR DISORDER 84
Dr Navin Nair Narayanan

CHAPTER 17 OVERVIEW OF SCHIZOPHRENIA 88
Dr Navin Nair Narayanan

CHAPTER 18 BIOAVAILABILITY OF VITAMIN D_3
             AND OMEGA 3 FATTY ACIDS 93
Dr Nomina Binti Ahmad Bustami

REFERENCES 97

CHAPTER 1

INTRODUCTION TO VITAMIN D_3

1. INTRODUCTION

Cholecalciferol and calcitriol

Vitamin D_3 (cholecalciferol) is a steroid which is produced in skin on exposure to sunlight (UVB rays). It has multiple physiological roles that are not confined to just the brain. Vitamin D_3 is an inactive substance which is then converted in the liver by hydroxylation into 25-hydroxy vitamin D_3 25 (OH) D, which is a stable circulating form of vitamin D_3. The 25(OH) D is later converted in the kidneys and in the brain through a second hydroxylation into an active form of vitamin D_3 that is known as, 1-α-25-dihydroxy Vitamin D_3 1, 25 $(OH)_2 D$ or calcitriol[1].

Existing evidence indicates that vitamin D_3, a neuroactive steroid, acting on the GABAergic system and plays a role in mood regulation amongst other actions[1]. Some indicators that point to vitamin D_3 being involved in neurological functions are that there are receptors for vitamin D_3 as well as enzymes that produce active form of D_3 present in the brain[2, 3].

Vitamin D_3 is also known to be involved in multiple functions at cellular level. Research has implicated many ways in which vitamin D_3 could also affect the developing human brain through its effects on synthesis of neurotransmitters, antioxidant effects, cell differentiation, neurotrophic factor expression, regulation of cytokines, intracellular calcium signaling, as well as gene expression involved in neuronal maturation, morphology and metabolism[4]. The active form of vitamin D_3, calcitriol or 1, 25 (OH)$_2$ D has a structure of a steroid and has endocrine, paracrine and autocrine effect[5]. 1, 25 (OH)$_2$ D has also been shown to affect neurotrophins[6]. Vitamin D_3 has been associated with reductions in brain Ca^{2+} levels[7]. 1, 25 (OH)$_2$D may also modulate $GABA_A$ in the brain in a similar fashion to other neuroactive steroids[8].

2. SOURCES OF VITAMIN D3

The main source of vitamin D in humans 80 to 90% is de novo synthesis from 7-dehydrosterol which occurs under the skin with the help of ultraviolet UVB that has a wavelength of 290 nm to 315 nm[5,6]. The remaining part of vitamin D is supplied through food such as small fish. Hence we see that vitamin D3 comes from two sources, namely production in the lower layers of skin and diet in the form of cholecalciferol.

Vitamin D_3 from these two sources are in an inactive form and needs to be activated through a two-step hydroxylation. 7 –dehydrocholesterol is a zoostrol that can be converted to cholecalciferol in the skin with the help of ultraviolet rays from sunlight. It is a provitamin of vitamin D3. Vitamin D_3 is also thought to be synthesized in the nervous system, regulating neuronal activities and exerting neuroprotective effects[9].

3. NORMAL SERUM LEVELS OF VITAMIN D3

Vitamin D_3, has a required daily allowance (RDA) of 600 IU/d for ages 1–70 years and 800 IU/d for the age group of 71 years and above, which corresponds to a serum level of 25-hydroxyvitamin D level of at least 20 ng/mL (50 nmol/L). This RDA for vitamin D was based on the presumption of minimal sun exposure taking into consideration the wide variability in vitamin D synthesis in the skin from ultraviolet light[10]. The circulating levels of 25-hydroxyvitamin D or 25 (OH) D are measured when estimating vitamin D_3 levels. Serum values of >30 ng/mL or 75 nmol/L, are required to maximize vitamin D's beneficial effects for health[11]. Vitamin D deficiency has been defined as serum 25(OH) D levels of <50 nmol/L. Sunlight appears to have greater effect on vitamin D_3 levels in men compared to women[12]. Deficiency or borderline level of vitamin D_3 is fairly common in the general population and may occur in almost one billion people on earth[5].

That is one billion of the seven and a half billion people who inhabit earth.

4. PREVALENCE OF DEFICIENCY

Recommended serum levels of 25(OH) D: are >30 ng/mL or 75 nmol/L.

- In a study done in USA on 18,875 subjects, 57% had levels less than 62.5 nmol/L[13]. This is less than the 75 nmol/L that has been suggested for optimum health.
- In another study, 36% out of the sample aged 18 to 29 years had hypovitaminosis[14].
- In Europe, the prevalence of deficiency of vitamin D_3 in the general population was 28–87% of the adult population[15]. The lowest concentration of 25 (OH) D due to season is usually observed during winter and spring[10].
- A study done on 316 young adults aged 30-50 years from the Middle East showed that 72.8% had 25(OH) D values of less than 15 ng/m L. This was in the severely low range and was possibly due to the attire worn in that part of the world which covers up most of the body[16].
- The prevalence of vitamin D deficiency was 33% amongst school children in Malaysia[17.] The mean vitamin D level was lower in females (53 ± 15 nmol/L)[17].

- A total of 858 participants were recruited for a study carried out in Malaysia. Subjects consisted of mainly Malay females. The prevalence of vitamin D deficiency (<20 ng/mL) was 67.4 %[18]. Also patients with higher body mass index were noted to have lower levels of vitamin D_3[18].
- A Malaysian study by Sadat-al et al on 1361 students (mean age 12.9±0.3 years) which consisted of 61.4% girls, showed deficiency in vitamin D in 78.9% of the participants. The deficiency was significantly higher in girls (92.6%, p<0.001), Indian adolescents (88.6%, p<0.001) and urban-living adolescents (88.8%, p<0.001). Hence female adolescents with greater waist circumference and those living in urban areas had higher risks of being vitamin D deficient. Serum 25(OH) D concentrations in that study were classified based as follows, 5<12.5 nmol/L=severely vitamin deficient; <37.5 nmol/L=vitamin D deficient; between37.5 and 50 nmol/L=vitamin D insufficient; ≥50 nmol/L=sufficient vitamin D[19].

CHAPTER 2

VITAMIN D_3 AND COGNITION

1. EFFECT OF LOW SERUM LEVELS OF VITAMIN D3 ON COGNITION

Low plasma vitamin D levels were associated with greater odds of cognitive impairment[11]. The relationship between 25(OH) D concentration and cognitive function was most pronounced at 25(OH) D concentrations below 35 nmol/L[20].

In the study by Lee et al 2009, 3,133 men (mean (+/-SD) age 60+/-11 years) were studied. The mean (+/-SD) 25(OH) D concentration was 63+/-31 nmol/L. High levels of 25(OH)D were associated with high scores on the copy component of the Rey-Osterrieth Complex Figure (ROCF test), the Camden Topographical Recognition Memory (CTRM)test and the Digit Symbol Substitution Test (DSST)[20].

Low levels of vitamin D_3 have been associated with impairment in cognition[21,22,23] In a study by Wilkins et al on 80 participants, vitamin D deficiency was associated with worse performance on the short blessed test (SBT)[21]. This is a test that can screen for dementia. Two studies by Przybelski and Chei show serum levels of 25(OH) D positively correlate with Mini Mental State Examination (MMSE)[22,23]. In another study on 1766 adults aged 65 years and older from the Health Survey for England 2000, which is a nationally representative population-based study, cognitive impairment was assessed using the Abbreviated Mental Test Score and correlated with D_3 levels. Data suggests that low serum 25(OH) D was associated with having increased odds of cognitive impairment[24]. In the study by Buell on more than a 1000 elderly individuals, serum 25(OH) D was positively associated with cognitive performance, particularly with measures of executive function. Further prospective studies are needed to examine the causal direction of the association[25]. In the Rancho Bernado study, vitamin D insufficiency was associated with poorer baseline performance on the MMSE, Trails Making Test B, Category Fluency, and Long Term Retrieval. It has been noted that even moderately low vitamin D was associated with poorer performance on multiple domains of cognitive function[26]. Cross-sectional studies cannot prove temporal relationships between serum levels and cognitive decline. It must be emphasized here that the onset of dementia itself might cause vitamin D concentrations through behavioral and dietary changes[27]. **Summarizing, vitamin D_3 levels are positively correlated with cognitive function.**

SPECIFIC ABNORMALITIES CAUSED BY VITAMIN D_3 ON COGNITION

1) Both depression and Alzheimer's disease display an increase in Ca^{2+} that has been linked to vitamin D deficiency[28,29].
2) Ca^{2+} acts to stimulate the formation of $A\beta$ plaques that are the hallmark of Alzheimer's dementia[30,31].

CHAPTER 3

VITAMIN D$_3$ AND DEPRESSION

MAJOR DEPRESSION@UNIPOLAR DEPRESSION

There are a few facts that suggest that vitamin D$_3$ plays a role in the genesis of depression.

1) Research shows that vitamin D deficiency is associated with an 8–14% increase in the risk of depression [32,33,34,35]. Specifically, low levels of serum 25(OH) D have been associated with depressive symptoms[35]. However replacing vitamin D$_3$ was not associated with amelioration of depressive symptoms according to multiple studies [36,37,38,39,40].

2) Also regular methods of treating depression with antidepressants are frequently of limited effectiveness[41]. Khoraminya et al. compared the therapeutic effects of fluoxetine, with and without vitamin D$_3$, in major depressive disorder, and showed significantly more improvement in depression scales for patients who received supplemented of vitamin D$_3$[10].

3) Receptors for calcitriol are found in almost all cells. In 1982, the presence of vitamin D$_3$ receptors were noted in the CNS[42], Brain structures involved in emotion and mood regulation such as cingulate cortex, hippocampus, thalamus, hypothalamus were

reported to have D_3 receptors[2]. The pathogenesis of depression is due to multiple factors and one of the factors could possibly be deficiency of vitamin D_3[43].

DYSFUNCTIONS CAUSED BY LOW LEVELS OF VITAMIN D_3 DURING DEPRESSION

The exact pathophysiology of depression is unclear. Vitamin D appears to be involved in multiple ways with respect to the onset and maintenance of depression.

1) **Vitamin D_3 is thought to act by reducing the increased neuronal levels of Ca^{2+} that are precipitated by depression.**

    The increase in neuronal Ca^{2+} levels has been hypothesized to be a major factor responsible for initiating the onset of depression[44]. The increased glutamate that occurs during depression increases Ca^{2+} through the activation of N-methyl-D-aspartate receptor (NMDAR) Ca^{2+} channels[44]. Vitamin D is able to maintain the Ca^{2+} pumps that reduce Ca^{2+} levels within the neuron, which may explain how it plays a role in reducing the onset of depression[44]. During hypovitaminosis this will not be possible and calcium levels will remain elevated in the cell.

2) **Activation of the expression of tyrosine hydroxylase.**

    The mood disorder is associated with deficiency in dopamine, noradrenaline and adrenaline. Calcitriol activates the expression of tyrosine hydroxylase, which is involved in the synthesis of these neurotransmitters, thus increasing the production of dopamine, noradrenaline and adrenaline[45]. However low levels of calcitriol will not be able to adequately activate production of the neurotransmitters.

3) **Vitamin D increases antioxidant activity in the brain.**

Vitamin D_3 increases the synthesis of gamma-glutamyl transpeptidase the enzyme which participates in the synthesis of glutathione which functions as an important antioxidant in the brain[46]. Antioxidants are needed to negate the effects of free radicals caused by oxidative stress. Oxidative stress occurs when there's an imbalance between free radical activity and antioxidant activity. In depression or chronic psychological stress there is increased oxidative stress with free radicals release. Antioxidants such as glutathione help to neutralize free radical activity and minimize damage to body tissues. Glutathione is involved in the disposal of peroxides by brain cells and in the protection of brain cells against reactive oxygen species. Prolonged free radical activity in the brain can lead to diminished hippocampal size as well as Alzheimer's disease, Parkinson's disease and many other neurodegenerative diseases.

4) **Vitamin D has anti-inflammatory action in the brain.**

- The pro inflammatory cytokines interleukin-1α and β, tumor necrosis factor-α (TNF-α), and interleukin-6 have been implicated in the onset of depression[47]. One of the important actions of vitamin D is to reduce inflammation through reducing the expression of inflammatory cytokines especially interleukin 6[48].
- Plasma level of tryptophan, an essential amino acid that is required for the synthesis of serotonin is decreased during inflammation[49].
- The increase in reactive oxidation stress (ROS) that occurs during inflammation is thought to induce depression through a number of ways such as an alteration in the formation of neurotransmitters such as serotonin and an increase in Ca^{2+} signaling.

Cytokines and the associated increase in ROS formation inhibit serotonin synthesis[50]. The increase of ROS also elevates intracellular Ca^{2+} levels by inhibiting the plasma membrane Ca^{2+}-ATPase (PMCA) pump on the plasma membrane that is critical for maintaining low resting cytosolic Ca^{2+} ($[Ca^{2+}]_i$) in all eukaryotic cells[51].

Summarising, vitamin D_3 appears to play multiple roles in the onset and maintenance of depressive states. Serum 25(OH) D levels are low in depressive states but its replenishment does not appear to attenuate depressive symptoms.

DEPRESSION IN THE ELDERLY

Depressive symptoms are more prevalent in older people, occurring in 8-16 % of persons over 55 years of age[52]. Vitamin D inadequacy is set at serum 25(OH) D levels of <50 nmol/L and occurs in about 50 % of elderly persons from Western countries[53].

Vitamin D deficiency affects especially women, who live in moderate climate countries due to a reduced amount of vitamin D containing food such as small fish in their diet and reduced amount of 7-dehydrocholesterol[10]. This reduced intake leads to diminished synthesis of vitamin D_3. Other causes of vitamin D deficiency in older persons include decreasing ability of the skin to produce vitamin D, a reduced amount of sun exposure and possible poorer absorption[54]. This lower level are associated with various adverse health outcomes, such as a greater risk of cardiovascular diseases[55], hospitalization and death[56] and reduced quality of life[57]. Treatment of depression in older persons is often not optimal, due to stigma by older generation, adverse effects of anti-depressant medication, or interactions of antidepressants with other medications[58]. Hence, development of a simple and safe prevention strategy is pivotal. Past research suggests that vitamin D supplementation may improve both mental and physical health, although evidence is inconsistent[59].

Results are mainly conflicting as to whether vitamin D supplementation does or does not improve depression in the elderly[60]. In a study by Alavi et al on 78 adults aged over 60 years with moderate to severe depression, subjects were randomly allocated to receive 50,000 U vitamin D_3 pearl weekly for 8 weeks or placebo. The main outcome measures comprised Geriatric Depression Scale-15 (GDS-15) questionnaire and 25(OH) D levels. Findings indicated that vitamin D supplementation was able to improve depression score in those aged 60 and over[59]. A study carried out by Milaneschi et al suggest that hypovitaminosis D is a risk factor for the development of depressive symptoms in older persons[60].

EFFECTS OF LOW LEVELS OF VITAMIN D_3 ON POST PARTUM WOMEN

We see that low levels of vitamin D not only has an undesirable effect on the mood of healthy adults but also the elderly population. In addition it affects pregnant women and women in confinement as well.

Postpartum depression (PPD) is a common disorder that affects 10–15% of women who recently delivered a baby, and it can have deleterious effects on both the mother and baby. Studies have suggested that low levels of vitamin D are associated with poor mood and depression. Lower serum vitamin D_3 levels during pregnancy were identified as a risk factor for development of postpartum depression[61]. Women in the study by Robinson reported postnatal depressive symptoms three days after delivery. Participants who scored in the lowest quartile for 25(OH)D status had higher chance to report a higher level of depression symptoms than women who were in the highest quartile for vitamin D levels. This was the result even after taking into consideration a range of confounding variables including season of birth, body mass index and sociodemographic factors. Low vitamin D during pregnancy is a risk factor for the development of postpartum depression symptoms[61]. Results of a systematic review by Aghajafari et al. indicates a significant association between vitamin D status and both antenatal as well as postnatal depression[62].

In another study by Hassan et al which compared vitamin D serum levels of a group of pregnant women who suffered a miscarriage compared with a group that did not, the 1st trimester, results show the mean level of serum vitamin D_3 for a miscarriage group was 17.3ng/dl, while for uneventful 1st trimester group was 30.5ng/dl[63]. While miscarriage as an adverse event is not directly related to mood, it can indirectly contribute to depression.

CHAPTER 4

VITAMIN D$_3$ AND BIPOLAR DISORDERS

MANIA

Vitamin D deficiency was 4.7 times more common among outpatients with bipolar disorder, schizophrenia, or schizoaffective disorder than among the Dutch general population[64].

ABNORMALITIES NOTED IN THE BRAIN DURING A MANIC EPISODE

1) **Increased intracellular calcium in bipolar disorder**

   We now know that vitamin D deficiency causes increased intracellular calcium. There is increasingly strong evidence for calcium signaling dysfunction in bipolar disorder[65]. There is a large amount of evidence from many studies implicating Ca$_V$ genes in the pathophysiology of psychiatric disorders. Many risk loci for psychiatric disorders fall within genes that encode for voltage-gated calcium channels (CaVs)[66]. Calcium that enters through CaVs is essential for several neuronal processes[66]. There is research underway targeting Ca$_V\alpha_1$, Ca$_V\alpha_2\delta$, and Ca$_V\beta$ subunits as possible therapeutic modalities to treat bipolar disorders. At present several drugs utilizing $Ca_V\alpha_1$, $Ca_V\alpha_2\delta$ subunits already exist, however these drugs are being used to treat cardiovascular conditions, pain, and epilepsy[66].

Calcium channel blockers such a nimodipine, verapamil and diltiazem targeting Ca_V1 channels are prescribed to treat cardiovascular conditions. Lamotrigine, a drug that blocks $Ca_V2.3$ channels, is now approved used to treat bipolar disorder[67,68].

2) Increased levels of vitamin D binding protein (DBP) in those with bipolar disorder

Another finding among bipolar patients is the identification of increased levels of vitamin D binding protein (DBP) in participants with bipolar disorder (BD) compared to non-mood control population. The increased levels of vitamin DBP in the circulation of adolescents with BD could be explained in two ways: DBP plays a role in the pathophysiology of BD in adolescents or DBP is a factor associated with this disorder. DBP levels in BD participants were significantly higher than in participants without any major mood disorders[69].

DBP effects multiple functions namely vitamin D binding protein help in transportation of vitamin D[70]. As little as 1–2% of DBP are bound to vitamin D. This implies that that DBP function may extend beyond its vitamin D transport properties[71]. The other functions of DBP include binding with fatty acids[70], extracellular structural protein[71], and trombospondin[72] and being in the circulation after cell necrosis and tissue injury. The carboxy-terminal domain of DBP also contains an O-linked glycosylation site. Enzymatic cleavage of this side transforms DBP into a lower molecular weight DBP-L[73]. This DBD-L has been redesignated as a strong macrophage-activating factor (termed DBP-MAF)[74]. The significance of DBP modifications to major mood disorders pathogenesis remains unknown.

3) **Decreased serum vitamin D levels in bipolar disorder**

In another study by Cuomo on 290 hospitalized patients, 272 patients (94%) showed vitamin D inadequacy. Of these 290 patients 243 had a diagnosis of bipolar disorder. Levels of physical activity and regular diet were positively correlated with vitamin D levels while advancing age, tobacco use, parathyroid hormones and alkaline phosphatase levels were negatively correlated[75]. In a study by Altunsoy et al contributed to the idea that vitamin D deficiency and acute manic episode may have interactions with many pathways. It has been recommend that serum vitamin D levels should be measured in bipolar patients especially over the extended period[76].

4) **Increased synthesis of vitamin D in the plasma during acute episode of mania.**

A study by Naifar has shown that acute episode of BD was accompanied by increased synthesis of plasma 25 (OH) D[77]. These results need to be replicated in other studies to be perceived as significant.

Summarizing, serum 25(OH) D levels are low in bipolar and it is suggested that serum levels may be monitored over the long term.

CHAPTER 5

VITAMIN D$_3$ AND SCHIZOPHRENIA

More than 50 million people worldwide have been diagnosed with schizophrenia[78]. It is one of the most disabling and costly chronic medical conditions because treatment-resistant symptoms are frequent[79]. Schizophrenia is a highly destructive illness as it strikes the young and is characterized by recurrent relapses, cognitive decline, emotional and functional disability[80]. Persons with this disorder frequently don't complete their schooling and are unable to hold jobs despite being on treatment. This symptoms of this disorder can be divided into positive symptoms such as hallucinations, delusions, negative symptoms such as emotional blunting, apathy and cognitive impairment. Negative symptoms and cognitive impairments are generally resistant to antipsychotic medication[81].

Recently there has been an impetus to consider what impact nutrition may have on mental disorders[82]. In addition, metabolic disturbances including insulin resistance and disordered lipid metabolism are related to cognitive impairment in schizophrenia which might help to retard functional decline found in these patients [83]

Psychological medicine is at a stage, where the current model which is mainy focused pharmacologically has achieved only modest benefits in solving the burden of poor functioning of these patients. Although the etiology of mental disorders are not well understood, there is emerging and compelling evidence that nutrition might be as important a factor to psychiatry as it has been found to be to other medical disciplines.

Evidence is steadily mounting for the relationship between vitamin D_3 deficiency and occurrence of schizophrenia, and for the use of nutrient-based supplements or lifestyle modifications to address these deficiencies. We have divided the research on vitamin D_3 deficiency into prenatal and postnatal periods as it appears to have effects prior to birth.

RESEARCH FOCUSSONG ON VITAMIN DEFECIENCY IN THE PRENATAL PERIOD.

Firstly we will elaborate on that research that was conducted on the prenatal period. Experiments on animals have shown that even a transient vitamin D deficiency during the prenatal period is associated with persistent changes in brain morphology and neurotrophin expression. In order to understand the effect of the vitamin D animal model of schizophrenia Becker et al examined different types of learning and memory in adult rats that were subject to transient prenatal vitamin D deficiency. When compared to the control rats, the prenatally deficient rats had a significant impairment of latent inhibition, which also happens to be found in schizophrenia[84].

Eyles et al. discovered that babies born with a vitamin D deficiency had a 44 percent higher risk of developing schizophrenia later in life. Also, this deficiency in newborns could account for about 8 percent of all schizophrenia diagnoses in Denmark[85]. Hence preventing vitamin D_3 deficiency in women who are pregnant, may therefore also prevent childrens' later risk of schizophrenia[85].

There is also evidence showing that low vitamin D_3 status during brain development in utero may contribute to the genesis of schizophrenia[86,87]. Mc Grath et al suggests that through analytic epidemiology, biological plausibility and assay development, genomics, proteomics and cellular neuroscience it has been shown that vitamin D plays a role in the development of schizophrenia.

In addition Berger has suggested that abnormal maturation of grey matter has been suggested as a partial explanation of early and late neural developmental abnormalities common in psychosis[88].

RESEARCH FOCUSSING ON VITAMIN D DEFECIENCY IN THE POST NATAL PERIOD

1) Normal vitamin D_3 levels decreases risk of schizophrenia.
2) Vitamin D deficiency associated with higher level of positive symptoms.
3) Vitamin D deficiency associated with higher level of negative symptoms.
4) Vitamin D deficiency associated with higher level of cognitive symptoms.
5) Vitamin D deficiency associated with higher level of depressive symptoms.
6) Vitamin D deficiency associated with poorer metabolic profile.
7) Supplementation with vitamin D_3 in the schizophrenic patient

There is a vast amount of research highlighting the prevalence of vitamin D_3 deficiency among chronic schizophrenics[89]. Many studies have found lower levels of vitamin D_3 in schizophrenic patients comped to normal controls[90-92].

In the study by Berg et al on Norwegians with psychosis, many psychotic patients had lower serum levels of 25 (OH)D than Norwegian in the reference sample that consisted of the general public[93]. Grados et al observed deficient vitamin D_3 levels in all the patients studied, being significantly lower for schizophrenic patients as compared to other psychoses[94]. More studies are required to examine in detail this association in schizophrenia because vitamin D_3 deficiency is easily remedied in an inexpensive manner by encouraging more sunlight exposure.

Another study by Berg researched the associations between vitamin D_3 levels and brain volume in patients with psychotic disorders that also takes into account possible interaction with genetic polymorphisms[95].

Vitamin D_3 levels were found to be significantly and positively associated with peripheral grey matter volume in patients. Also a more rapid rate of cortical grey matter decline has been consistently found in persons who convert from a high risk of psychosis to frank psychosis and this phenomenon has been attributed to neuro inflammation[96].

1) **Normal vitamin D_3 levels decreases risk of schizophrenia**

A study carried out by Hakko et al on 9114 subjects to ascertain the association between the use of vitamin D supplements during the first year of life and risk of developing schizophrenia showed that in males, the use of any type of supplementation either irregular or regular vitamin D supplementation was associated with a reduced risk of schizophrenia[97]. In the first year of life, data was collected regarding the frequency and dose of vitamin D supplementation. Vitamin D supplementation during the first year of life is associated with a reduced risk of schizophrenia in males. Hence it was concluded that preventing hypovitaminosis D during early life may reduce the incidence of schizophrenia. Similarly in a study carried out by Valipour et al. on vitamin D deficient participants showed they were 2.16 times more likely to develop schizophrenia compared to vitamin D non deficient participants[89].

Vitamin D deficiency can lead to dysfunction of the hippocampus—a brain region hypothesized to be critically involved in schizophrenia. In the study by Shivakumar et al, potential association between serum vitamin D level and hippocampal gray matter volume in antipsychotic-naïve or antipsychotic-free schizophrenia patients (n = 35) was examined. Serum vitamin D_3 level was calculated using 25-OH vitamin D immunoassay. A significant and positive correlation was seen between vitamin D and regional gray matter volume in the right hippocampus after controlling for age, years of education and total intracranial volume. These observations support a potential role of vitamin D deficiency in mediating hippocampal volume deficits, possibly through neurotrophic, neuro-immunomodulatory and glutamatergic effects[98].

Cieslak et al carried out a study to assess the Leukocyte Telomere Length (LTL), a marker of cellular aging with vitamin D levels in

22 well-characterized schizophrenia cases to assess if the association was spurious or caudal. The patients were examined with respect to symptoms, cognition, and functioning. The results showed that 91% (20) had deficient or insufficient vitamin D levels, and this was associated with excitement and grandiosity, social anhedonia and poverty of speech. Gender specific analyses showed strong associations of hypovitamintosis D to negative symptoms and decreased premorbid adjustment in males, and to lesser hallucinations and emotional withdrawal, but it was associated with increased aggression in females[99].

2) **Vitamin D deficiency associated with higher level of positive symptoms**

In the study by Bulut when patients with and without vitamin D deficiency were compared, it was found that there was a statistically significant difference between their SANS and SAPS total scores as well as of the some subscale scores, such as affective flattening, bizarre behavior, and positive formal thought. At greater levels of vitamin D deficiency, higher scores on the SANS and SAPS scales were obtained. Of the schizophrenic patients who participated in this study, 61.25% were found to have adequate levels (>20 ng/mL), 20% showed deficient levels of vitamin D< 10 ng/mL and 13.75% were found to have insufficient level 10-20 ng/mL As a result of vitamin D deficiency, positive symptoms such as disorganized speech and disorganized behavior and cognitive symptoms of attention and memory deficit were noted[100].

3) **Vitamin D deficiency associated with higher level of negative symptoms**

Yee et al. found an association between low bioavailable vitamin D and negative symptoms in first episode psychosis (FEP) in Singapore[101]. To our knowledge, only two other studies have examined the correlation between vitamin D and psychotic and/or affective symptoms in FEP. Graham et al. found that greater severities of negative symptoms are correlated with lower vitamin D levels but not with depressive or overall symptoms in first-episode schizophrenia patients in North Carolina, USA[102].

4) Vitamin D deficiency associated with poorer cognition

Vitamin D deficiency is thought to cause memory and attention deficits by reducing GABAergic and glutamatergic neurotransmissions, which are important for attention and working memory in the dorsolateral prefrontal cortex. Therefore, vitamin D deficiency could theoretically also lead to reduced dorsolateral dopaminergic transmission, which may lead to attention and memory deficits[103]. Vitamin D's close relationship to the dopaminergic system has been documented[104].

In a study by Bulut that included 80 patients diagnosed with schizophrenia and 74 age-and sex-matched controls, the Scale for the Assessment of Negative Symptoms (SANS) and the Scale for the Assessment of Positive Symptoms (SAPS) were used to assess the symptom severity. It was found that there was a negative correlation between 25(OH) D levels and SANS total points; a negative correlation for attention points and negative correlation with positive formal thoughts. The results of this study show a relationship between lower levels of vitamin D and the occurrence of positive and negative symptoms[100].

Another study by Krivoy showed that Vitamin D supplementation was associated with an improved cognition, however it did not affect psychosis or mood[105].

5) Low vitamin D_3 levels is associated with higher levels of depressive symptoms in schizophrenia.

There is a strong association between low 25(OH) D and higher negative and depressive symptoms in psychotic disorders[106].

6) Vitamin D deficiency associated with poorer metabolic profile

Probiotic together with vitamin D for 12 weeks administered to chronic schizophrenics had beneficial effects on the general and total

PANSS score, and metabolic profiles. Vitamin D and probiotic co-supplementation also significantly increased total antioxidant capacity, and significantly decreased malondialdehyde and high sensitivity C-reactive protein levels compared with the placebo. It was also noted that, taking vitamin D plus probiotic significantly reduced fasting plasma glucose, insulin concentrations, triglycerides and total cholesterol levels and total-/HDL-cholesterol ratio[107].

Recent studies have suggested a potential role of vitamin D_3 in the development of schizophrenia. For example, neonatal vitamin D_3 status is associated with the risk of developing schizophrenia in later life. Obesity, insulin resistance, diabetes, hyperlipidaemia and cardiovascular disease, are commonly seen in patients with schizophrenia[108]. It has been well established that vitamin D_3 deficiency is related to these metabolic problems. The biological mechanism is most likely related to vitamin D's action on the regulation of inflammatory and immunological processes, consequently affecting the manifestation of clinical symptoms and treatment response of schizophrenia.

7) Supplementation with vitamin D_3

Patients in an acute episode had significantly lower vitamin D levels compared to patients in remission and to healthy controls[109]. It is not known if vitamin D deficiency is the result or the cause of an acute episode. The idea that vitamin D deficiency and schizophrenia may have interactions with an unknown pathway has been suggested. Present data points out a possible influence at a genomic level. Serum vitamin D levels should be measured in patients with schizophrenia especially in long term care. Further treatment with add-on vitamin D supplements and diets that are rich in vitamin D should be considered.

Up until 2013 no study had had investigated the potential psychotropic effects of vitamin D supplementation in patients with psychosis.[110]. A study by Hendoiee et al added vitamin D to the standard therapeutic regimen of schizophrenic male patients with inadequate vitamin D status in order to assess if it could improve some aspects of the symptom burden. Eighty patients with chronic and stable schizophrenia having only residual symptoms and vitamin D deficiency were recruited randomly and then received either 600000 IU Vitamin D injection once along with their antipsychotic regimen or with their antipsychotic regimen only. Serum vitamin D was measured twice: initially at baseline and repeated on the fourth month. Positive and Negative Syndrome Scale (PANSS) was assessed at both occasions. In vitamin D and control group there was a negative but insignificant correlation between serum vitamin D level changes and PANSS negative subscale score. The authors did not find any relationship between serum vitamin D level changes and the improvement of positive symptoms in schizophrenic patients and suggested more randomized clinical trials are required to confirm their findings[111]. However there is increasing evidence suggesting that vitamin supplementation, in particular with folic acid, vitamin B12 and vitamin D, may be important in treatment within certain subgroups of patients. This review also reiterated the need for research with larger samples before any conclusions can be made[112].

Summarizing, serum 25(OH) D levels are low in schizophrenic disorders. Vitamin D supplementation in pregnancy may play a preventive role in schizophrenia occurrence. Finally, serum 25(OH) D levels should be monitored in schizophrenic patients, especially those who are on long term care. At present there is no conclusive evidence that supplementation of vitamin D ameliorates psychopathology.

CHAPTER 6

INTRODUCTION TO OMEGA 3

1. INTRODUCTION

Polyunsaturated fatty acids (PUFA) consists of omega 3, 6 and 9. Omega-3 fatty acids, is one of the main components of cell membranes[113]. Omega-3 fatty acids, also called omega-3 oils, ω–3 fatty acids or n–3 fatty acids, and they are characterized by a double bond three atoms away from the terminal methyl group in their structure[113]. Three types of omega–3 fatty acids involved in human physiology are alpha linolenic acid (ALA), found in plant oils and hormones, and eicosapentaenoic acid (EPA) and docosahexaenoic acid (DHA), both commonly found in fish oils[114].

DHA is thought to act by increasing the fluidity of cell membranes compared to other PUFAs. Fluidity of membranes determines the site and activity of membrane proteins, including enzymes, ion transporters, and receptors of neurotransmitters[115].

From their site on membrane phospholipids, EPA and DHA are released by phospholipases on the cue of various stimuli. EPA acts as a precursor to eicosanoids. Eicosanoids are signaling molecules made through enzymatic or non-enzymatic oxidation of EPA. Subfamilies of ecosanoides are prostaglandins, thromboxanes, and leukotrienes regulating inflammation, vasomotion and hemostasis[116]. Arachidonic acid (a type of omega 6 fatty acid) derivatives are pro-inflammatory, whereas eicosanoids derived from EPA are relatively antiinflammatory[116]. Hence this is why our body needs adequate amounts of omega 3.

Although EPA exists in substantially lower concentrations than AA, increased EPA availability competes with, and reduces the production of, AA-derived eicosanoids.

There is some evidence that omega-3 fatty acids are related to mental health and also that they may possibly help as add-on treatments for depression associated with bipolar disorder[117]. Obvious benefits due to EPA supplementation were only seen, when treating depressive symptoms suggesting a link between omega-3 and low mood[116]. This connection between omega-3 and depressive disorders has been thought to be due to the fact that many of the products of the omega-3 synthesis pathway play important roles in decreasing inflammation which have been linked to depression[119] This connection to inflammation regulation has been supported in both in vivo studies and in a meta-analysis[120].

There is some evidence of positive effect on mild cognitive problems, especially mild Alzheimer's dementia[121]. DHA-rich supplementation has been shown to be less effective than EPA-abundant supplementation in enhancing neurocognitive functioning after a 30-day supplementation. Epidemiological studies do not conclude if omega-3 fatty acids has any beneficial effects on the mechanisms of Alzheimer's disease. LC omega-3 PUFA are also postulated to ameliorate behavioral and mental health disturbances in schizophrenia and attention deficit hyperactivity disorder[119].

2. SOURCES OF OMEGA 3

Omega 3 comes from plants and animals[113]. Our source of omega 3 comes from both exogenous and endogenous sources. Exogenous refers to plant and animal sources. Endogenous sources refers to conversion of ALA to DHA and EPA. Between the two omega fatty acids it is said that DHA is the more important one for cognition and EPA for depression.

ALA is a plant source of omega 3. Both marine algae and phytoplankton are primary sources of omega-3 fatty acids[113]. Sources of plant oils containing ALA include nuts such as walnut, cauliflower, flaxseed oil and hemp oil, while sources of animal omega-3 fatty acids EPA and DHA include fish especially salmon, tuna, sardine, mackerel, anchovies, fish oils, eggs from chickens fed EPA and DHA, squid oils, krill oil, and some types of algae[114]

Human beings are unable to synthesize much essential omega-3 fatty acid and can only get it through food[122]. However, once in the body, the liver can convert ALA, to form EPA and DHA, by creating extra double bonds along its carbon chain and elongating[122]. Namely, ALA (18 carbons and 3 double bonds) is used to make EPA (20 carbons and 5 double bonds), and later used to make DHA (22 carbons and 6 double bonds). DHA can also be a substrate for the genesis of EPA and vice versa[123] However this being said the efficiency of conversion of ALA to EPA is very poor, less than 5%[122]. In humans, approximately 1 % of DHA may be retroconverted to EPA[119] Hence it is imperative to take adequate exogenous omega 3. Based on isotope tracer experiments it is indicated that overall conversion of ALA to DHA in man appears to be very low at 0.5% to -4 %[119].

It is obvious that there exists a competition between the omega-6 and omega-3 fatty acid families for metabolism, since the both pathways use the same enzymes. The preferred substrate for D6 -desaturase is ALA, but the relative excess of linolenic acid (LA) in our diet means that the pathway involving omega-6 fatty acids prevails[119]. Tissue levels of the omega-6 and omega-3 PUFAs and their corresponding eicosanoid metabolites link directly to the amount of dietary omega-6 versus omega-3 PUFAs consumed. Some of the omega-6 and omega-3 PUFA metabolites have almost diametrically opposing physiological and pathological actions, hence it has often been said that the deleterious consequences associated with the consumption of omega-6 PUFA-rich diets causes excessive production and activities of omega-6 PUFA-derived eicosanoids.

Generally, the omega-3 fatty acid nutrition amongst Malaysians is not adequate and far from desirable[122]. The nutritional situation with respect to long-chain polyunsaturated fatty acids (LCPUFA) amongst Malaysian pregnant and lactating women is alarming and warrants urgent action in nutrition promotion activities/counselling[122]. A study done in Malaysia showed that the various sources of omega-3 fatty acids in the Malaysian diet are edible oils (ALA), fish its products (EPA+DHA), vegetables (ALA), meat and eggs (EPA+DHA), and milk and its products (EPA+DHA) and that Malaysians could still meet the daily requirements by eating a balanced diet[124].

Omega-6/ omega-3 fatty acid ratios are in the region 8-11:1[122]. We tend to eat too much omega-6 fatty acid with little attention paid to omega-3 fatty acid nutrition. A study done in Malaysia on staff and medical students obtained a ratio of omega-6/omega-3 FA ratio of >20: 1, which is very unsatisfactory compared with the WHO recommendation of 5-10: 1.4[122]. A lower omega-6/omega-3 fatty acid ratio, should be emphasized with respect to increased omega-3 fatty acid intake[122]. That means we need to eat more foods that are rich in omega 3.

3. NORMAL SERUM LEVELS OF OMEGA 3

The dose of omega 3 ranges from 1000 to 2000 mg per day.[125] Some even recommend 3000 mg per day of EPA and DHA. Most Americans and much of the developed world consume less than 200 mg per day of EPA and DHA[126]. The daily dose requirement can go up to 2.6 g in pregnant and lactating women[125]. For DHA the recommended dose for this population is 100 to 300 mg daily[122].

Essential fatty acids (EFA) are called as "essential" and must be supplied by the diet. There are two such essential fatty acids. The two EFA being **linoleic acid** (LA which is an omega 6 fatty acid) and the second one often consumed in much smaller quantities is **alpha-linolenic acid** (ALA which is an omega 3 fatty acid). LA is metabolized to the 20-carbon arachidonic acid (omega-6), while ALA which is from vegetable sources is metabolized to the omega-3 long-chain polyunsaturated fatty acids (LCPUFA) EPA and DHA.

Studies have tested a daily dose of 1 gram omega-3 supplementation and found there is wide interpersonal variation in blood omega-3 levels achieved in response to a fixed daily dose[127]. Omega-3 blood level ranges may vary due to environmental and genetic reasons[127].

Different eating habits predispose to different interactions between food fatty acids. Omega-3 acids are susceptible to oxidation, and their storage conditions often lead to a dramatic increase in oxidation. Therefore, the effect of oxidation on their bioavailability needs also to be considered.

Attention must be paid to effective methods of supplementation. Bioavailability addresses both the speed of absorption and the amount of the fatty acids absorbed[114]. The speed can be interpreted as how fast the fatty acid is absorbed from the gastrointestinal tract and reaches the portal system. Absorption of the fatty acid occurs in the gastrointestinal tract to some extent. This depends on multiple factors. The extent of absorption and the speed of substance transport to the portal circulation describe the bioavailability of the fatty acid.[114].

4. Deficiency

A deficiency of essential fatty acids—either omega-3s may predispose to rough, scaly skin and dermatitis[128]. Plasma and tissue concentrations of DHA can become lower when there is poor omega-3 fatty acid intake[128]. However, there are no known cut-off levels of DHA or EPA below which there are neural or visual impairment or immune response, becomes affected.

Supplementing the brain with DHA has been considered as therapy for the DHA brain deficiency that could be associated with neuronal death or neurodegeneration. The human brain has, a compensatory mechanism for loss of neurons in the brain called neurogenesis which is the production of neurons derived from stem cells. In adults, neurogenesis still continues, albeit at a slower rate and with lower efficiency[129].

Emergence of cerebral diseases also can occur with low omega 3 levels. Dietary intake of omega-3 PUFA could not modify neurologic disturbances associated with aging or neurodegenerative diseases. As decreased levels of DHA have been associated with degenerative diseases of the brain, targeting the brain with DHA might hold great promise in developing new strategies for neurodegenerative diseases[129]

CHAPTER 7

OMEGA 3 AND COGNITION

EFFECTS OF SUPPLEMENTATION ON VARIOUS POPULATION GROUPS

It is thought that omega 3 can prevent dementia. 47.5 million people worldwide have dementia and with 7.7 million new cases[130]. Prevention of dementia can be brought about through diet. There is growing body of evidence showing that certain nutritional factors could be associated with cognitive impairment (CI)[131]. Omega 3 PUFAs are thought to play an important role in the prevention of dementia[132]. Other supplements thought to play a role in the prevention of dementia are, Vitamin E, B vitamins, folates, and Ginkgo biloba[133].

Bauer et al, has shown that an increase in EPA intake is more advantageous than DHA in reducing "effort" relative to cognitive performance. Brain imaging has been known to show consistent changes in neurochemicals, electrical activity, cerebral metabolic activity and oxygenation of brain after omega-3 supplementation[134]. In another study by Bauer et al, it was concluded that following the EPA-rich supplementation, patients' brains worked 'less hard' and achieved a better cognitive performance than before supplementation[135].

PUFA have shown improvements in all ages of people with respect to cognition. In a study on school going children living in the United

States, PUFA intake was associated with better attention and working memory performance[136].

The grey matter of the brain contains high levels of DHA. Although the role of DHA in the developing brain and in dementia has attracted much attention, its influence on the brain of the healthy adult has been little explored. DHA supplementation has been shown to improve memory and the reaction time of memory in healthy, young adults whose habitual diets were low in DHA[137]. Omega-3 supplementation is associated with an improvement of attentional and physiological functions, particularly those functions entailing complex cortical processing[137].

In another study on women Omega-3 Index (O3I) was used to determine the percentage of EPA and DHA in the red cell membrane, and the sample was divided into four groups: T1 < 5.47%, T2 = 5.47–6.75%, T3 > 6.75%. Potentially confounding factors of BMI, inflammatory status, physical activity, alpha1-acid glycoprotein, serum ferritin and hemoglobin, were assessed. Attention domain of cognition was poorer in women with lower O3I, however it was still considered normal. This reduced but normal level of cognition potentially provides a lower baseline from which cognition would deteriorate with advancing age[138].

Randomized clinical trials (RCTs) suggest that enhancing the diets of both to be mothers and infants with DHA improves cognitive development[139].

Supplementation with omega-3 PUFA did not show any benefit in the cognitive function in institutionalized elderly people who did not have cognitive impairment[140]. However a larger set of studies has reported findings in the elderly, where the sample studies had a mean age exceeding 55 years. Of these, three cross-sectional studies were available in which the investigators tested associations between self-reported fish intake and cognitive performance assessed with multicomponent neuropsychological batteries. Subjects whose mean daily intake of fish was >/=10 g/d, had significantly better mean test scores and a lower prevalence of poor cognitive performance than did those whose intake was poor i.e <10 g/d. These associations between total intake of seafood and cognition were very much noted to be dose-dependent. The majority of cognitive functions were influenced by fish intake. This phenomenon was more pronounced for non-processed lean fish and fatty fish[141].

As we know cognition encompasses a variety of function in the brain. PUFA are said to favorably affect certain functions like psychomotor speed. Kalmijn et al found evidence that fish intake is primarily related to psychomotor speed rather than episodic memory and mental flexibility[142]. Many studies have found that EPA and DHA supplementation improved memory, psychomotor speed, and prepotent response inhibition. Stonehouse et al found evidence of performance improvement on tests of episodic and working memory with a DHA supplement that varied with gender[137]. Omega-3 supplementation has been associated with an improvement of attentional and physiological functions, particularly those involving complex cortical processing[143]. Significant intervention effects for specific performance domains were unfortunately not consistently observed and the majority of statistical comparisons were null[142]. This being said, Jackson et al found no notable beneficial effects from either DHA-rich or EPA-rich supplementation[144].

Dosing is also of significance. In the United States, dietary intake of the long-chain omega-3 PUFAs averages110 mg per day[125], and supplementing 400 mg daily increases circulating levels by 50%[145]. Two studies on affective disorders found some benefits from 1,000 mg per day of EPA per day with no incremental benefit from higher doses[146,147]. Some studies employing doses under 800 mg per day generally found no treatment effects[144].

A number of RCTs have found that fish oil supplementation is efficacious in patients with attention deficit disorders[148]. In summary there has been much research done with respect to omega 3 and cognition. **Summarizing benefits of omega with respect to cognition, omega 3 specifically DHA appears to improve attention, processing speed and seems to have some effect in most age groups, and in addition it may prevent dementia.**

CHAPTER 8

OMEGA -3 FATTY ACIDS AND DEPRESSIVE DISORDERS

There has been long debate as to whether there is any difference between EPA and DHA in treating depression. Also it is not known if omega 3s initiate their effects on depression differently or synergistically. EPA and DHA play different roles in depression because of their different involvement in anti-inflammatory activity and their maintenance of membrane integrity and fluidity[149]. According to Deacon et al the treatment efficacy of supplementation with omega-3 PUFAs in depression is influenced by the proportion or dosage of EPA or DHA[149].

It currently felt that EPA is more superior compared to DHA, in treating depression. Hence people with depression should choose a combination that is higher in EPA. A study done by Liao et al showed that omega-3 PUFAs with EPA ≥ 60% at a dosage of ≤1 g/d has beneficial effects on depression[150]. According to the study by Liao et al DHA-pure and DHA-major treatments failed to show significant efficacy in alleviating depression, while EPA-pure and EPA-major treatments were beneficial in improving depression[150]. PUFAs that mainly consists of EPA (EPA > 50%[151], 60%[152], and 80%[153] of the dose) have significantly greater efficacy than those that are mainly DHA (DHA > 50%, 60%, and 80% of the dose, respectively), regardless of PUFAs monotherapy or adjuvant use. Recent double-blinded randomized controlled trials (RCTs) indicated that EPA, mostly at dosages of 1 or 2 g/d, was better than placebo and DHA as a monotherapy or adjuvant in the treatment of mild to moderate depression and that the ratio of an 'active' synergetic effect between EPA and DHA would probably be either 2:1 or 3:1 [154,155] Mischoulon et al also reported that compared to 4 g/d, greater efficacy was found at 1 g/d and 2 g/d in a single-arm randomized trial on depression [155]. The effect that EPA can decrease depression was concordant with those of previous studies and may be mediated by the known mechanism at the cellular level [156, 157].

MECHANISMS BY WHICH EPA AND DHA EXERT ANTIDEPRESSANT EFFECTS.

Since EPA levels are highly correlated with inflammation, EPA supplementation might benefit only major depressive disorder (MDD) subjects with inflammation as part of their syndrome and that it may even be potentially harmful for individuals whose MDD was due to a different physiological disturbance [150]. Also we cannot determine whether the efficacy occurs because of EPA itself or because of an interaction with DHA supplementation. Some possible mechanisms of EPA and DHA are demonstrated below.

EPA can easily enter the brain as a free fatty acid and is not reacylated into phospholipid membrane stores because it is quickly metabolized and oxidized [159]. Based on this process its contribution to anti-inflammation in depression has been extensively documented, and both DHA and EPA or EPA alone may reduce the occurrence of inflammation due to eicosanoids such as prostaglandins, leukotrienes and thromboxanes [160].

1. ANTIINFLAMATORY EFFECTS

There are a few ways that omega 3 fatty acids can decrease inflammation.

a) In the first instance, DHA and EPA can lead to a decrease in production of pro-inflammatory cytokines, such as interleukin (IL)-1β, IL-2, and IL-6, which have also been associated with depression[161].

b) Secondly, both DHA and EPA can reduce inflammation through combining with arachidonic acid (AA) by incorporation into membrane-based phospholipids, causing a decline in both cellular and plasma concentrations of AA[150]. AA is a type of omega 6 fatty acid which produces pro inflammatory substances hence reduced levels of AA will yield less inflammatory substances.

c) The other possibility is that EPA, but not DHA, can bring down the production of AA by inhibiting delta-5-desaturase activity[150]. Gamma linolenic acid can be converted to AA by the enzyme delta-5-desaturase.

d) EPA may compete with AA for phospholipase A_2 (PLA_2) and prevent the process of pro inflammatory eicosanoid synthesis from AA. These pro inflammatory eicosanoids are known as prostaglandins, thromboxanes, and leukotrienes[158]. **Essentially, AA is responsible for inflammation in the body and omega-3 can decrease AA which is a pro inflammatory substance.**

2. NEUROPROTECTION

a) EPA SUPPLEMENTATIN INCREASES N-ACETYL-ASPARTATE

EPA supplementation has been associated with N-acetyl-aspartate(NAA) increases in the brain, which is a marker for neuronal homeostasis, suggesting its role as a neuroprotective agent[162]. NAA is a nervous system-specific metabolite, which is occurs in neurons and appears to be a key link in biochemistry of CNS metabolism. During initial postnatal CNS development, there is increased NAA production in neurons. NAA is transported from neurons to the cytoplasm of oligodendrocytes, to be made into fatty acid and steroids. The fatty acids and steroids then go on to be used as substrate for myelin lipid genesis. Once postnatal myelination is completed, NAA may continue to play a part in myelin synthesis in adults[163].

NAA can also be used for energy production in mitochondria. NAA also is said to play a role in the production of mitochondrial energy from glutamate[163].

NAA can act as a magnetic resonance spectroscopy marker for the state of neuronal health, viability and number. Evidence suggests that NAA is a direct precursor for the enzymatic synthesis of, dipeptide N-acetylaspartylglutamate the most concentrated neuropeptide in the human brain. Other proposed roles for NAA include neuronal osmoregulation and axon-glial signaling[163]. Hence we can say that NAA is an important substance in the brain.

b) EPA SUPPLEMENTATION INCREASES BRAIN DERIVED NEUROTROPHIC FACTOR

Nerve growth factors (NGF) was discovered in the early 1950s and discovered to have trophic effects on sensory and sympathetic neurons. In 1982, brain-derived neurotrophic factor (BDNF), the second member of the "neurotrophic" family of neurotrophic factors, was shown to help in the survival of dorsal root ganglion neurons[166]. EPA supplementation has been shown to increase brain-derived neurotrophic factor (BDNF) levels after traumatic brain injury[165,166].

In addition to BDNF playing an important role in neuronal survival and growth, it also serves as one of the neurotransmitters, and increases neuronal plasticity, which is essential for learning and memory. BDNF is widely found in the CNS and gut. BDNF and insulin-like growth factor-1 have similar downstream signaling mechanisms that promote survival genes. BDNF regulates glucose and energy use. Decreased levels of BDNF have been associated with many degenerative diseases of neuronal loss, such as Parkinson's disease, Alzheimer's disease, multiple sclerosis and Huntington's disease. Hence, BDNF may be useful in the prevention and management of several diseases[167].

3. NEUROTRANSMITTER

Benefits of EPA may be partly related to its ability to increase dopaminergic and serotonergic neurotransmission[168]. Long chain marine omega-3 fatty acids in the brain consist primarily of the C22 n-3 DHA with some C20 n-3 EPA[169].

EPA INCREASES SEROTONIN RELEASE.

Omega-3 fatty acids can modulate serotonin function through regulation of serotonin release in the presynaptic neuron. Serotonin release is normally inhibited by prostaglandins which are generated from AA[170,171]. EPA inhibits the formation AA which in turn results in no or less production of prostaglandins[172,173]. With the resulting lowered amounts of prostaglandins, more serotonin is released. One of the evidence for this increased release of serotonin is that omega 3 serum levels have been positively correlated with the serotonin metabolite, 5-hydroxy indole acetic acid (5-HIAA) levels in cerebral spinal fluid[174]. This means that since greater amounts of serotonin were released in to the synaptic cleft as the inhibitory effects of the prostaglandin were removed, this resulted in higher levels of serotonin metabolite i.e 5-HIAA in the body.

Serotonin

Serotonin is an important neurotransmitter in the brain and is concentrated in brain regions known to regulate social cognition, decision-making as well as maintaining normal mood. Evidence links serotonin to social behavior as well[175,176]. Polymorphisms in the serotonin transporter gene have been linked to social behavioral defects including violence, impulsivity, anxiety disorders, and other psychopathology such as antisocial personality[177]. As we know the gene codes for the protein, in this case the protein is serotonin.

Lowering brain serotonin levels in normal people leads to many behavioral consequences such as impulsive behavior, problems learning, poor memory, poor long-term planning, inability to resist immediate gratification, and social behavioral deficits characterized by impulse aggression or not being altruistic[176].

DHA influences development and maintenance of dopaminergic neurons.

DHA is one of a number of ligands for the nuclear receptor RXR. In the dopaminergic system,

4. DHA INCREASES MEMBRANE FLUIDITY

DHA has been proposed to influence serotonin effects by increasing membrane fluidity and thus serotonin receptor accessibility is increased in postsynaptic neurons[179]. Also, DHA fluidity of membranes modulates the location and activity of membrane-bound proteins, including enzymes, ion transporters, and neurotransmitter receptors[115].

Serum levels of EPA and DHA have been found to be low in those with a wide range of psychiatric illnesses including autism spectrum disorder (ASD), attention deficit hyperactivity disorder (ADHD), bipolar disorder, schizophrenia, cases of parasuicide, and those with impulsivity. Supplementation has been shown to have a beneficial role in modifying the severity of symptoms of these disorders.

Suicidal ideation is common in patients treated for bipolar disorder and depression and has been linked to both low omega-3 and low serotonin in the brain[181,182]. Randomized controlled trials have found that supplementation with several grams of EPA and DHA improved depression, suicidal thoughts, and behaviors[180,183]. **Of late, meta-analyses show a clear benefit for omega-3 fatty acids in the treatment of depression however there is some heterogeneity between clinical trials**[184,185]. Reasons for inconsistent results in the studies include genetic variation between participants, types of omega-3 fatty acid from diet and different EPA and DHA ratio and dose in various formulations[186,187]. Many people do not get enough omega 3 fatty acids as evidenced in this study where dietary surveys in the United States have shown that the average adult intakes of linoleic acid (omega-6 fatty acid), ALA (omega-3 fatty acid), EPA, and DHA are :-12–20, 1.4–2.0, 0.03–0.06, and 0.05–0.10 g/d, respectively[188].

Summarizing the role of omega 3 in depressive disorders, it appears that EPA plays a bigger part than DHA in alleviating mood. EPA acts through its multiple anti- inflammatory mechanisms, neuroprotection (increasing NAA and BDNF) as well as increasing neurotransmitter (serotonin and dopamine) levels.

DHA meanwhile influences serotonin effects by increasing membrane fluidity and thus serotonin receptor accessibility is increased especially in postsynaptic neurons.

Chapter 9

OMEGA 3 AND BIPOLAR DISORDER

Bipolar disorder is a chronic, debilitating and recurrent illness with significant impairment in functioning[189]. Bipolar it most commonly start during the adolescence[189]. Causative factors are thought to be are having bipolar disorder in family history, various forms of abuse, other psychosocial stressors, substance use disorders, psychostimulant and antidepressant medication exposure and last but not least omega-3 fatty acid deficiency[189].

Prodromal mood symptoms generally precede the onset of mania by an average of 10 years, hence interventions initiated prior to onset of the disorder should be safe and well tolerated to cater for prolonged exposure[189]. Constituents of prodromal symptoms include episodic symptoms of depression, anxiety, hypomania, in appropriate anger/irritability and sleep disruptions and poor attention[189] Antidepressant as well as psychostimulant medications may trigger the onset of mania[189]. Mood stabilizers and atypical antipsychotic medications are efficacious in youth with bipolar I disorder, however not much is known about the efficacy of these medications during prodrome[189].

Omega-3 fatty acids possess neurotrophic and neuroprotective characeristics and have been found to be efficacious, safe and well tolerated in the treatment of manic and depressive symptoms in both children and adolescents alike. It is believed that omega-3 fatty acids are a potential treatment for bipolar disorder because the fish-oil fatty acids, EPA and DHA, can alter brain signal pathways in ways similar to mood stabilizers like lithium and valproate[189]. DHA has multiple roles in the body. DHA has been shown to promote neuronal survival[190] and differentiation[191] in both transformed and primary neuronal cells in culture. Considering the fact that astroglia support neurons by providing neurotrophic factors, DHA supplied by astroglia may also be trophic[192]. Numerous studies have indicated that this concentration of DHA in the nervous system is essential for optimal neuronal and retinal functions.

Long-chain polyunsaturated fatty acids are found in abundance in the nervous system. Docosahexaenoic acid (DHA; 22:6 n-3), in particular, is the most abundant polyunsaturated fatty acid in the brain and is found in concentrated form in aminophospholipids of cell membranes[193]. It is well established that DHA can be biosynthesized from alpha-linolenic acid (18:3 n-3), a shorter chain-3 fatty acid precursor, through chain elongation and desaturation processes. Alpha linolenic acid is desaturated to 18:4n-3 by 6-desaturase, chain elongated to 20:4n-3, and subsequently converted to eicosapentaenoic acid (20:5n-3) by5-desaturase in the endoplasmic reticulum[193]. The precursor fatty acid ALA (18:3n-3), found in vegetable oils acts partly as a source of energy and partly as a precursor of the metabolites, but the degree of conversion appears to be severely restricted. Most studies in humans have shown that though restricted, conversion of high doses of ALA to EPA does occur, but conversion to DHA is severely restricted. The use of ALA labelled with radioisotopes shows that with a diet high in saturated fats, conversion to long-chain metabolites is approximately 6% for EPA and 3.8% for DHA. When we ingest a diet rich in omega-6 PUFA, conversion is further reduced by 40 to 50%.

DHA can be released readily from astroglial membranes under basal and stimulated conditions, and supplied to neurons[194].

Postmortem examinations of bipolar patients have found significantly lower DHA concentrations in the prefrontal cortex compared with the general population, and epidemiological surveys have found that people who eat more fish or seafood are less likely to have bipolar disorder[195]. Epidemiological and biochemical studies demonstrate convincing evidence regarding the relationship between bipolar disorder and reduced consumption of omega-3. In general, low levels of omega-3 in the blood and brain tissue after death have been found in bipolar patients. There is no definitive explanation yet, but lack of omega-3 consumption appears to be a preventable risk factor for recurrent mood disorder[196]. In a study by a researcher, McNamara in the United States of America, the relationship of omega-3 fatty acids with mood disorders and their effects on the prevention and treatment of these disorders was studied. The results showed that omega-3 can contribute to reduce the symptoms of these patients and also reduces their suicide rates[197].

Omega-3 supplement was effective for the treatment of BD, it is suggested to use omega-3 supplements as an adjuvant therapy along with the other pharmacotherapies[198]. The gradual diminishing in structural and functional integrity of brain tissue appears to correlate with loss in membrane DHA concentrations. Arachidonic acid, also predominant in this tissue, is a major precursor for the synthesis of eicosanoids that act as signaling mechanisms. Aging predisposes to a likely increase in reactive oxygen species and hence a concomitant decline in membrane PUFA concentrations, and with it, cognitive impairment.[199]

Neurodegenerative disorders such as Parkinson's and Alzheimer's disease also appear to exhibit membrane loss of PUFAs. Hence supplementation with n-3 fatty acids may help to delay their onset or reduce the insult to brain functions which these diseases elicit[199].

Evidence suggests mechanisms for PUFAs in BD. Omega -3 PUFAs seem to be an effective adjunctive treatment for bipolar depression, but larger-scale, well-controlled trials are needed to examine its clinical utility in BD. The use of omega-3 as a mood stabilizer among BD patients has been suggested[200]. This article summarizes the molecular pathways related to the role of omega-3 as a neuroprotective and neurogenic agent, with a specific focus on BDNF[200b]. It is proposed that the omega-3 BDNF association is involved in the pathophysiology of BD and represents a promising target for developing a novel class of rationally devised therapies 200. This study by Safari et al aimed at assessing the effect of omega 3 as compared with fluvoxamine in the treatment of depression in bipolar patients[201].

Research findings related to the effects of omega-3 was found to be harmless. It is suggested that omega3 can be prescribed with other anti-depressive medicines. Prior studies have shown that fatty acid supplementation may be useful for unipolar depression, but the data has been more mixed for bipolar disorder. People with bipolar disorder have lower levels of certain omega-3 fatty acids that cross the blood-brain barrier compared to those who do not, according to researchers.

Summarizing role of omega in bipolar disorder, the evidence endorses a model in which subjects at elevated risk for developing mood disorder may be treated with safe interventions such as omega-3 fatty acids and family-focused therapy in the prodromal phase[189].

CHAPTER 10

OMEGA 3 AND SCHIZOPHRENIA

The biological mechanisms underlying any beneficial effects omega-3 LC-PUFAs on the brain are currently unknown and need to be investigated. Omega-3 LC-PUFAs have proven to be indispensible with regards to neural development and function. As key components of brain tissue, omega-3 PUFAs play important roles in brain development and function, and a lack of these fatty acids has been implicated in a number of mental health disorders and this list encompasses schizophrenia.

Over the last 10 years many studies were carried out assessing the feasibility of early detection of people at risk of developing psychosis and interventions to prevent or delay a first onset psychotic episode. Unfortunately most of these studies were small and underpowered[202]. A meta-analysis[202] demonstrated the effectiveness of PUFA to prevent or postpone a first episode of psychosis. In the study by van der Gaag a search conducted identified 10 studies reporting 12-month follow-up data on transition to psychosis, and 5 studies with follow-ups varying from 1 to 2 years. Early detection and intervention in people at ultra-high risk of developing psychosis can be successful to prevent or delay a first psychosis[202].

When focusing on just EPA, the meta-analysis that included 167 patients treated with EPA and 168 who received placebo found no benefit in EPA supplementation for people with established schizophrenia. EPA supplementation may be preventative for pre-psychotic populations and also may alleviate extrapyramidal and metabolic side effects of antipsychotic[203].

The identification of an ultra-high risk (UHR) profile for psychosis and a greater understanding of its prodrome have led to increasing interest in early intervention in intercepting the onset of psychotic illness[204-206]. Amminger et al have conducted a few studies showing that long chain omega-3 PUFAs have a preventive role in transitioning to psychosis[204]. A reputable randomized, double-blind, placebo-controlled study that included 81 adolescents and young adults of ages 13 to 25 who were at significantly higher risk of developing schizophrenia compared to the general population were administered either 1.2 g/day of omega-3 fatty acid or placebo for 12 weeks, and subsequently monitored for 40 more weeks. The omega-3 group showed moderate to large effects in that only two omega-3-treated subjects became psychotic as compared to eleven in the placebo group. In contrast to antipsychotics, the effects of omega-3s persisted beyond treatment and are considered safer than antipsychotics, particularly for adolescents and children[204].

Another similar study was a randomized, double-blind, placebo-controlled trial, carried out with a follow up of 6.7 years. Here brief intervention with omega-3 PUFAs reduced both the risk of progression to psychotic disorder and psychiatric morbidity in general in this study. The majority of the individuals from the omega-3 group did not show severe functional impairment and no longer experienced attenuated psychotic symptoms at follow-up[205]

While PUFAs are well tolerated and seem to be of help in prevention of psychosis, they are not effective in alleviating symptoms of schizophrenia. Outcomes of using PUFAs to treat tardive dyskinesia or extra-pyramidal symptoms are inconclusive. A review by Mossaheb et al examined multiple studies regarding the use of PUFAs in treating psychosis. Maybe the ratio of omega-3s to omega-6s might be more important than absolute values. They concluded that while they are generally not effective in treating established schizophrenia, PUFAs may be preventative to those susceptible to schizophrenia[206].

In a randomized placebo-controlled trial, by Smesny et al the authors identified a long-chain omega-3 PUFA supplementation as potentially useful, as it reduced the rate of transition to psychosis by 22.6% 1 year after baseline in a cohort of 81 young people at ultra-high risk of transition to psychosis. In this paper, the authors also reported on the effects of omega-3 PUFA supplementation on intracellular phospholipase A_2 (inPLA$_2$) activity, the main enzymes regulating phospholipid metabolism, as well as on peripheral membrane lipid profiles in the individuals who participated in this randomized placebo-controlled trial. Patients were studied cross-sectionally ($n=80$) and longitudinally ($n=65$) before and after a 12-week intervention with 1.2 g per day ω-3 PUFAs or placebo, followed by a 40-week observation period to establish the rates of transition to psychosis. The authors investigated inPLA$_2$ and erythrocyte membrane FAs in the treatment groups (omega-3 PUFAs vs placebo) and the outcome groups (psychotic vs non-psychotic). The levels of membrane omega-3 and omega-6 PUFAs and inPLA$_2$ were significantly related. Supplementation with omega-3 PUFA resulted in a significant decrease in inPLA$_2$ activity. The authors concluded that omega-3 PUFA supplementation may act by normalizing inPLA$_2$ activity and δ-6-desaturase-mediated metabolism of omega-3 and omega-6 PUFAs, suggesting their role in neuroprogression of psychosis[207]. This being said, the mechanisms whereby the omega-3 PUFAs might be neuroprotective are not well understood.

Omega-3 fatty acids most probably can prevent the development of full-blown schizophrenia in people who are at high risk of the disease. There is a growing increasing evidence that omega-3 fatty acids can prevent schizophrenia or at least mitigate the course and symptoms. Appropriate dietary supplementation may be able to contribute a partially therapeutic effect, even in more severe patients, improving some behavioral aspects and, mainly, reducing the cognitive deterioration[208].

In addition to prevention of transition to psychosis, omega 3 has been known to have other benefits on schizophrenia such as on negative symptoms. A statistically significant negative correlation was reported between omega-3 fatty acids and negative symptoms in the never-medicated[209]. That means the higher the omega levels are, the less the negative symptoms.

These benefits of omega -3 extend to cognition as well. In a study by Satgomi et al the results of 30 patients indicated that decreased serum omega-3 fatty acids are correlated with cognitive impairment, which in turn impacts social functioning outcomes in schizophrenia[210]. Cognitive impairment is strongly associated with functional outcome in patients with schizophrenia but its pathophysiology is unclear. Effects of omega-3 fatty acids in the cognitive function of healthy individuals and patients with neuropsychiatric disease gets a lot of attention. Polypharmacy often used to treat schizophrenia also has been shown to affect cognition[211].

Violent schizophrenic patients treated with fish oil (360 mg DHA + 540 mg EPA) demonstrated a decrease in violence, but improvement in positive and negative symptoms was no greater than patients treated with the placebo after twelve weeks[212]. For example, beneficial effects in mood disorders have more consistently been reported in clinical trials using EPA; whereas, with neurodegenerative conditions such as Alzheimer's disease, the focus has been on DHA[213].

During an acute episode of schizophrenia, patients with low RBC PUFA have more negative symptoms and more metabolic and haematological abnormalities than those with high PUFA. This may show that PUFA levels define two clinically distinct phenotypes of the disorder[214]. PUFA concentrations in erythrocyte membranes are decreased in schizophrenia. Of particular importance in patients are lower concentrations of DHA and AA, two fatty acids that are abundant in the brain and important precursors in the cell-signalling cascade[215].

Another abnormality noted in schizophrenia is an electrophysiological measure N400 of semantic memory and language that correlates with deficits in schizophrenia. Relationships among N400, cognition, dopamine, and cell membrane PUFAs were examined for in patients tested for those medicated with haloperidol only and placebo conditions[216]. Levels of total PUFAs and arachidonic acid were associated with N400 in un- medicated patients. Clinical symptoms such as paranoid delusions and disorganized thought but not cognition was associated with N400. These results suggest that fatty acids present in red cell membrane are associated with semantic memory and language in schizophrenia. Summarizing, omega-3 fatty acids is basically stigma-free and should be considered for use as a prevention against psychosis as it has minimal risks and side effects.

Summarizing the effects of omega-3 in schizophrenia, it can be said that it possibly has a preventive role during prodrome but no effect on frank psychosis. In addition it may improve cognition. Its effects on negative symptoms and violence needs to be studied further. Also as omega 3 has well established effects on depression, it would be good to assess if it can alleviate the low mood that often accompanies schizophrenia.

Chapter 11

INTRODUCTION TO MAGNESIUM

1. INTRODUCTION

Magnesium (Mg2+) is an essential ion in humans, playing a key role in supporting and sustaining a healthy body[217]. It is the fourth most common cation in the body and the second most commonly found intracellular cation next to potassium[217]. Magnesium takes part in more than 600 enzymatic reactions including energy metabolism and protein synthesis. Theodor Günther stated the number of enzymatic reactions as 300 using it as a rough estimate in 1980 and this has been in use ever since. However, in the years that followed after 1980 many new magnesium dependent enzymes have been discovered, and now we know that the number 300 is a huge underestimation of the true importance of magnesium. At present, enzymatic databases describe over 600 enzymes for which magnesium serves as cofactor, and another 200 in which magnesium may act as activator[218,219].

2. SOURCES OF MAGNESIUM

Dairy products, vegetables such as spinach and kale, fruits such as avocados, bananas and raspberries, salmon, mackerel, tuna and poultry are the main sources of dietary magnesium intake Over the last 60 years the magnesium content in fruit and vegetables decreased by 20–30%. Part of the problem originates from the soil used for agriculture, which is becoming increasingly deficient in essential minerals[230]. 80–90% of magnesium is estimated to be lost during food processing[217]. As a result, a significant number of people are magnesium deficient[217].

3. NORMAL SERUM LEVELS OF MAGNESIUM

Although magnesium availability has been proven to be disturbed during several clinical situations, serum magnesium values are not generally determined in patient[217]. Supplementation of magnesium is known to be beneficial in treatment of, depression, migraine preeclampsia, coronary artery disease, and asthma[217].

Magnesium deficiency is commonly determined by measuring total serum magnesium concentrations, which ranges between 1.5 to 1.9 m Eq/L in a healthy person[221]. A healthy human adult body has about 25 g or 1000 mmol Mg where approximately 60% are stored in bones, 20% in muscles, 20% in soft tissues, 0.5% in erythrocytes, and 0.3% in the serum[221]. This being said, serum magnesium values reflects at best only 1% of the body magnesium content, as most of the magnesium is stored in bone, muscle, and soft tissues. Hence despite serum values are within the normal range, the body may be in a severely magnesium -depleted state. Consequently, the clinical impact of magnesium deficiency may be largely underestimated. In a study on Malaysian aboriginals showed that serum magnesium levels for aborigines were 1.178 ± 0.221 mmol/l[222]. This was in the normal range.

4. PREVALENCE OF DEFICIENCY

Over the last ten years, several hereditary forms of hypomagnesemia have been discovered, including those due to mutations in transient receptor potential cation family melastatin type, claudin 16 which are major components of tight junctions, and cyclin M2. Magnesium plays a role in cell signaling, cell proliferation, enzymatic activity and nucleotide binding among other functons[217]. Hypomagnesemia can be the due to the use of some drugs, such as diuretics, epidermal growth factor receptor inhibitors, calcineurin inhibitors, and proton pump inhibitors[217].

Among adults in the United States of America, 68% consumed less than the recommended daily allowance of magnesium, and 19% consumed less than 50% of the RDA. After controlling for demographic and cardiovascular risk factors, adults who consumed <RDA of magnesium were 1.48-1.75 times more likely to have elevated C-reactive protein (CRP) than adults who consumed > or =RDA[223]. CRP is a protein that increases in the blood when there is inflammation somewhere in the body.

In a study by Galan et al on 5448 French subjects, cereal products represented the main contribution of magnesium in both men (21 per cent) and women (19.8 per cent). In the same study, the second source for men was represented by alcoholic beverages (11.7 per cent), but this constituted a lower source of magnesium in women (5.5 per cent). The overall mean dietary intake was estimated at 369 +/- 106 mg/day in men and 280 +/- 84 mg/day in women. 77 per cent of women and 72 per cent of men had dietary magnesium intakes lower than recommended dietary allowances. A strong positive correlation existed between energy and magnesium intake[224]. 72% of middle aged French adults have been shown to consume less than the recommended levels of dietary magnesium[224]. The United States Food and Nutrition Board recommends a daily intake of 420 mg for men and 320 mg for women[225] Research indicates that hypomagnesemia is associated with greater risk of mortality, sepsis, need for mechanical ventilation, and longer duration of ICU stay. Magnesium therapy for improving outcomes in critically ill patients is needed to further study.[226].

MAGNESIUM EFFECTS ON MENTAL ILLNESS

Magnesium plays multiple physiological roles in many organs namely brain, heart and muscles[217]. Magnesium is one of the essential mineral in the human body, and is connected with brain biochemistry and the fluidity of neuronal membrane. Many neuromuscular and psychiatric symptoms, including depressive states, has been observed in magnesium deficiency[227]. It is not fully understood yet how magnesium alleviates depression[227]. Magnesium treatment has been hypothesized to be effective in treating major depression resulting from intra neuronal magnesium deficits. Magnesium ions regulate calcium ion flow in neuronal calcium channels. In magnesium deficiency, neuronal requirements for magnesium are deficient, causing damage to the neurons which might manifest as depression. These magnesium ion neuronal deficits may also be induced by excessive intake of calcium, stress hormones, as well as dietary deficiencies of magnesium[228]. Magnesium supplementation seem to be an invaluable addition to the pharmacological management of depression[227]. 126 patients underwent 6 weeks intervention of active treatment (248 mg of elemental magnesium per day) compared to 6 weeks of control group who had no treatment at all. Assessments of depression symptoms were completed twice a week phone calls. Consumption of magnesium chloride for 6 consecutive weeks resulted in a clinically significant net improvement in depression and anxiety scores Average adherence was 83% by pill count[229]. These effects were observed within two weeks. Magnesium is effective for mild-to-moderate depression in adults. Case histories have shown rapid recovery that is, less than 7 days from major depression using 125–300 mg of magnesium in the form of glycinate and taurinate[228].

Treatment with magnesium supplements has been shown to induce rapid recovery from depression[230]. Depression has been associated with deficiencies of tryptophan, selenium, vitamin D, magnesium, and serotonin[231]. The correlation between tryptophan and other biomarkers/trace elements is also important in depression[231]. A review consisting of 20 articles by Ljungberg revealed that high adherence to dietary recommendations, avoiding processed foods, intake of anti-inflammatory diet, magnesium and folic acid, various fatty acids, and fish intake had a preventive effect on depression[232].

Magnesium has also been associated with subjective anxiety, leading to the proposition that its supplementation may decrease anxiety symptoms[233].

Vitamin D and magnesium supplementation in 66 children with ADHD[234] was shown to be effective on conduct and social problems as well as anxiety scores compared to placebo. Magnesium is known to reduce hyperactivity component in children with ADHD[235]. Patients with other mental illness like schizophrenia have lower erythrocyte magnesium levels than controls[236]. **Summarizing the beneficial effects of magnesium for mental health, supplementing magnesium in depression appears to have some positive effect. While supplementing magnesium appears promising with respect to depression more research is needed with respect to other mental illnesses.**

CHAPTER 12

INTRODUCTION TO FOLATE

1. INTRODUCTION

Folate otherwise known as folic acid is a water soluble B-vitamin involved in the synthesis, repair, and methylation of DNA. Folate plays an important part in maintaining mechanisms of DNA metabolism such as nucleotide synthesis[237]. Prophylactic antenatal intake of folic acid (FA) is said to reduce incidences of neural tube defects in infants. Folate has been extensively investigated for its unique functions as mediator for the transfer of one-carbon moieties for nucleotide synthesis as well as the repair and process of methylation. For the effective utilization of folate we need adequate daily intake of folate. Individuals who have either depression or schizophrenia have been known to have lower dietary folate intake as well as lower serum levels of folate.

Previously it was also suggested that folate supplementation improved the efficacy of traditional antidepressant medications. Future research on folate supplementation in depression is warranted and clinicians may consider L-methylfolate supplementation for patients suffering from depression or schizophrenia.

2. SOURCES OF FOLATE

Some sources of folate include leafy green vegetables, like spinach, broccoli, lettuce, beans, peas, and lentils, fruits like lemons, bananas, and melons, fortified and enriched products, orange juice, and bread, rice pasta, cereals

3. NORMAL SERUM LEVELS OF FOLATE

The reference range of the plasma folate level varies by age. In adults it is 2-20 ng/mL, 2-20 µg/L, or 4.5-45.3 nmol/L. While in children folate levels are in the range of 5-21 ng/mL, 5-21 µg/L, or 11.3-47.6 nmol/L. Serum folate is almost entirely in the form of N-(5)-methyl tetrahydrofolate[238].

Lower than normal serum folate also has been reported in patients with neuropsychiatric disorders, in pregnant women whose fetuses have neural tube defects, and in women who have recently had spontaneous abortions[239]. Folate deficiency is most commonly due to insufficient dietary intake, it is also frequently encountered in pregnant women or in alcoholics. Persistent alcohol consumption leads to deficiency of folate due to dietary inadequacy, intestinal malabsorption, decreased hepatic uptake and increased excretion. The decreased concentration of serum folic acid may occur in the majority of alcoholics.

The recommended daily amount of folate for adults is 400 micrograms (mcg). Adult women who are planning pregnancy or could become pregnant should be advised to get 400 to 800 mcg of folate a day[240].

It must be mentioned that while supplementation of folic acid may be conceived as beneficial it has been known to dysregulate expressions of several genes including FMR1 in lymphoblastoid cells, and a mouse model has also identified widespread alteration in the methylation pattern of the brain epigenome in offspring having high maternal folic acid during pregnancy. These alterations in the methylation pattern resulted in differences in the expression of several key developmental and imprinted genes. In addition it was noted that the methylation and expression of several genes were changed in a gender-specific manner. In future, more research on supplementation and over supplementation as well as their effects on epigenetic alterations will be needed so supplementation can occur without associated side effects.

Folate is also useful in non- psychiatric conditions. A dose-response meta-analysis indicated that a 100 μg/day increment in dietary folate intake reduced the estimate risk of esophageal cancer by 12%. These findings suggest that dietary and serum folate exert a protective effect against esophageal carcinogenesis[241].

A study by Saedisomeolia showed that folate deficiency is common in schizophrenic patients, therefore, it is important to pay attention to folate levels in these patients[242]. Certain people with hereditary deficits in their folate cycle metabolism have been found more likely to be schizophrenic than the general population. Babies born during famines are more likely to develop schizophrenia a few years later.

High folate ingestion can mask vitamin B 12 deficiency until neurological effects become irreversible. Detecting, treating, and preferably preventing, vitamin B-12 deficiency is vital especially in the current era of folic acid fortification. However this issue may be remedied by taking a supplement that contains 100 percent of the daily value of both folic acid and vitamin B 12 so that we do not end up treating folic acid deficiency and leaving the concurrent B 12 deficiency untreated.

FOLATE METABOLISM

MTHFR (methylenetetrahydrofolate reductase) an enzyme, activates folate in our diet into the active compound, 5 –methyl tetra hydro folate (5-methyl THF) to be used in the brain. Many people have a less efficient version of this enzyme. Genetic variants within the folate metabolic pathway can predispose one to negative symptoms of schizophrenia. There exists a relationship between negative symptoms severity and folate levels[243]

Polymorphisms in other genes such as, COMT and MTR gene which code for the enzyme methionine synthase also confer a higher risk of schizophrenia[243]. The study by Roffman et al showed that MTHRF 677T, MTR 2756A, FOLH1 484C and COMT 675 A predicted a greater negative symptom phenomenology in schizophrenia[243]. Negative symptoms in schizophrenia are described as disruptions in normal responses for a healthy individual and commonly include the inability to experience pleasure, disturbance of speech, flattened affect, and lack of motivation.

FOLATE AND METHYLATION

Methylation is a simple biochemical process whereby the transfer of four atoms i.e one carbon atom and three hydrogen atoms (CH3) occurs from one substance to another. When optimal methylation occurs, it has a significant positive impact on many biochemical reactions in the body that regulate the activity of the cardiovascular, neurological, reproductive, and detoxification systems, including those relating to neurotransmitter and DNA production. CH3 is provided to the body through a universal methyl donor known as SAMe (S-adenosylmethionine). SAMe easily donates its methyl group, which enables the cardiovascular, neurological, reproductive, and detoxification systems to perform their functions. Unfortunately, the system that produces SAMe is reliant on, 5-MTHF also known as active folate or methylfolate. When methylation does not occur then a number of important molecules cannot be efficiently produced, including norepinephrine, epinephrine, melatonin and serotonin. Deficiencies of the above neurotransmitters are seen in depression.

Methylene tetra hydro folate reductase (MTHFR)

MTHFR gene encodes for methylene tetra hydro folate reductase (MTHFR). MTHFR is the enzyme responsible for the formation of 5 –methyl tetra hydro folate (5-methyl THF) from dietary folate. 5-methyl THF allows conversion of homocysteine to methionine and adenosyl methionine by methionine synthetase (MTR) and is part of the AldoMet cycle[244]. Reduced MTHFR activity results in hyper homocysteinemia, which has been associated with coronary vascular disease.

Polymorphisms in MTHFR lead to a lack of 5-MTHF which interrupts methionine synthase activity. The two SNPs shown for MTHFR, C677T and A1298C have been shown to reduce MTHFR activity and thus lead to homocysteine accumulation.[245.]

This interruption leads to the accumulation of homocysteine and a reduction in the levels of methionine. Homocysteine is a marker of inflammation, when its levels in the body get too high it leads to the health issues. When less 5-MTHF is produced, less is available for methionine synthase to use in the conversion of homocysteine into methionine.

B12 is a cofactor for methionine synthase which re methylates homocysteine into methionine.

4. PREVALENCE OF DEFICIENCY

There are only a few studies on serum folate levels in the Malaysian populations. Most studies assessed folate levels with respect to neural tube defects (NTD) and in women at antenatal clinic or those of child bearing age.

In a study by Siew et al, the mean total intake of folates from diet was 260.281 g/d for males and 321.934 g/d for females. Chinese subjects tended to have significantly higher folate intakes 325.451 g/d compared to the Malay subjects 261.514 g/d. Analysis of food consumption showed that the folate intake was below the Recommended Nutrient Intake (RNI) for Malaysia 400 g/d. Most of the subjects had normal levels of serum folate, vitamin B12 and B6. However, the majority of the subjects were deficient in RBC folate and slightly more than half had elevated serum homocysteine levels[245].

In a study by Geok on 399 pregnant women, a 24-hour recall revealed that, the median intake level for folate was 202.4µg (59.4-491.8

μg) and this amounted to 50.6% of the Malaysian Recommended Nutrient Intakes level. The median (5-95th percentiles) values for plasma and red cell folate (RBC) concentrations were 11 (4-33) nmol/L and 633 (303-1209) nmol/L respectively. Overall, nearly 15.1% of the sample manifested plasma folate deficiency (< 6.8 nmol/L), with Indians having the highest prevalence (21.5%). Overall prevalence of RBC folate deficiency (< 363 nmol/L) was 9.3%, and it was an almost similar level prevailed for each ethnic group. Only 15.2% had RBC concentration exceeding 906 nmol/L[247].

According to Bailey et al normal serum folate levels are ≥ 6.8 nmol/L, deficient levels are ≤ 6.8 nmol/L, RBC folate normal levels are ≥ 363 nmol/L, deficient levels are ≤ 363 nmol/L, serum vitamin B12 normal levels are between 148–664 pmol/L, deficient levels are ≤148 pmol/L and serum vitamin B6 levels, normal is ≥ 20 nmol/L, deficient ≤ 20 nmol/L[248].

FOLIC ACID AND MENTAL ILLNESS

People suffering from mental illnesses like depression, schizophrenia, and dementia often have lower levels of serum folate compared to the healthy people[249].

Low folate levels are linked to a diminished response to antidepressants, and treatment with folic acid is shown to improve that response[250]. The use of folate preparations such as folic acid, folinic acid and L-methyl folate have proven to be effective at augmenting antidepressants in a variety of controlled and open-label settings in patients with normal and hypofolatemic status[250]. Research also suggests that high vitamin B12 levels may be associated with better treatment outcome in depression[251].

Folate and vitamin B12 are involved in one-carbon metabolism, in which S-adenosylmethionine (SAM) is formed. SAM donates methyl groups that are crucial for neurological function.

Increased serum levels of homocysteine is a functional marker of both folate and vitamin B12 deficiency[251]. Increased homocysteine levels are found in depressive patients. In a large population study from

Norway increased plasma homocysteine was associated with increased risk of depression but not anxiety. Furthermore, the MTHFR C677T polymorphism that impairs the homocysteine metabolism is shown to be overrepresented among depressive patients, which strengthens this hypothesis.

On the basis of current data, Coppen et al has recommended that oral doses of both folic acid at 800 μg daily and vitamin B12 at a dose of 1 mg daily should be used to improve treatment outcomes among those suffering from depression[251]. The utility of folate in mental illness has been known for several years, but the strategic use of L-methylfolate supplementation has not yet been accepted as a standard regimen anywhere[249]. Even the use of L-methylfolate as a monotherapy has been noted to possess antidepressant properties[249]. It has been suggested that we should consider the use of L-methylfolate as an adjunct to antidepressant medications[249].

With respect to schizophrenia, L-methylfolate supplementation was associated with physiologic changes with selective symptomatic improvement in schizophrenic patients,[252]. A study by Menegas et al has evaluated the efficacy of folic acid as a therapeutic adjunct to lithium on the manic behaviors as well as parameters of oxidative stress and inflammation in an animal model of mania induced by m-amphetamine. FA administration reduced the increased TNF-α content induced by m-AMPH. This study provides evidence that FA is effective as an adjunct to lithium standard therapy on manic-like behaviors, oxidative stress and inflammatory parameters in a model of mania induced by m-AMPH[253].

A study by Ma et al aimed to evaluate whether folic acid supplementation improved cognitive performance by reducing serum inflammatory cytokine concentrations. Findings suggested that, daily oral administration of a 400-μg folic acid supplement to mild cognitive impairment (MCI) subjects for a period of 12 months can significantly improve cognitive performance and reduce peripheral inflammatory cytokine levels[254].

Summary serum folate levels may be low in depression, schizophrenia and some dementias. Folic acid supplementation may improve antidepressant response and may act as an antidepressant itself. It may improve negative features in schizophrenia and has some benefit on cognition as well as animal models of mania.

CHAPTER 13

INTRODUCTION TO ZINC

1. INTRODUCTION

Zinc is the second most abundant divalent cation after calcium and is a component in hundreds of enzymes and proteins in the body and plays an integral role in over 300 biological processes.[255]. Zinc is an essential micronutrient that accumulates in brain in the glutamatergic neurons and is required for normal neuronal development and function[256]. Zinc participation is essential for neurotransmission[257]. Zinc is also required the processes of DNA replication such as transcription, protein synthesis, folding of proteins, maintenance of cell membranes, cellular transport, as well as endocrine and immunological systems.[258]. In addition zinc plays an important role as a cofactor in catalytic interactions and modulation ion channel activity[259].

The human brain contains significant amounts of zinc, with 5–15% concentrated in synaptic vesicles of glutamatergic neurons alone. Somas of the neurons that contain zinc are located in the cerebral cortex and in the amygdala, while their axons project towards the cerebral cortex and amygdala, striatum as well as structures of the limbic system. Zinc is packed into the synaptic vesicles by means of a zinc transporter 3 (ZnT-3), which is situated on the membranes of the vesicles. After the action potential it is released from the presynaptic vesicles into the synaptic cleft, there is no consensus as to the concentrations to which the zinc ion rises in the synaptic cleft. It is estimated to range from sub-μM to over 100 μM[260]. Zinc is said to be released into the synaptic cleft at concentrations ranging from from low doses in the region of nanomoles at rest to high micromoles during active neurotransmission[259].

Clinical, molecular, and genetic research show key roles for zinc homeostasis in association with clinical depression and psychosis[255]. Multiple well powered clinical studies have shown beneficial effects of supplementing zinc in depression and it important to engage in research that uses zinc as a potential therapeutic option for psychosis as well[255]. Meta-analyses support the adjunctive use of zinc in major depression and a study now supports zinc for psychosis amelioration[255].

2. SOURCES OF ZINC

Zinc is obtained from dietary sources, especially red meat, poultry, fish, and dairy products. Stringent regulation of zinc concentrations is essential as dietary intake of zinc varies as much as 15-fold. Its concentration is normally maintained by easy absorption in the digestive tract, but insufficiency can be related to poor diet, aging, medical comorbidities including alcoholism, H Pylori infections and the usage of numerous common medications such as antacids, diuretics, anticonvulsants, anti-retrovirals, hormones, steroids, anti-inflammatories, and cardiovascular medications. Zinc is present in all body tissues, having higher concentrations within muscle and bone.

3. SERUM LEVELS OF ZINC

Zinc is mostly protein bound and not in its free form with blood levels normally maintained between 80 to 100 µg/dL or 12 to 15 µmol/L[260]. The total body content of zinc in adults ranges from 1.5 to 2.5 g, with higher contents in males compared to women. Zinc is present in all organs, tissues, fluids, and secretions, but more than 95% is present in intracellular compartments. Intracellular deficiency may arise from low circulating zinc levels due to dietary insufficiency, or impaired absorption from old age, medical conditions, and alcohol dependence. Many medications commonly administered to psychiatric patients, such as antiepileptics, oral hypoglycaemic drugs, hormones, antacids, anti-inflammatories also affect zinc absorption[255].

4. PREVALENCE OF DEFICIENCY

In 2011, 1.1 billion people were at risk of zinc deficiency due to inadequate dietary supply[261]. Approximately 90% of those at risk of zinc deficiency in 2011 were from the continents of Africa and Asia[261]. Despite there being wide prevalence of zinc deficiency, a study on Malaysian aboriginals showed that serum zinc levels for aborigines were 15.847 ± 1.348 μmol/L / L[222]. This value was considered to be within the normal range.

Phytate, a substance that impairs zinc absorption and is the primary storage form of both phosphate and inositol in plant seeds[262]. Phytates form complexes with dietary minerals, especially iron and zinc, and lead to mineral deficiencies in people[262]. Phytates adversely affect protein and lipid utilization. This is a major concern for those individuals who are vegetarians as they can't get their zinc from meat[262]. Phytate consumption is useful to us in that it provides protection against a variety of cancers mediated through its antioxidant properties such as interruption of cellular signal transduction, cell cycle inhibition and enhancement of natural killer cells activity. Phytates also have therapeutic use against diabetes mellitus, atherosclerosis and coronary heart disease and reduces formations of kidney stones.

Processing techniques, such as soaking, germination, malting and fermentation, reduce phytates by increasing activity of naturally present phytase. Increased phytase activity leads to enhanced mineral absorption.

A study by Noraizan et al on the inhibitory effects of phytate on the bioavailability of iron, zinc and calcium assessed 29 food samples consisting of 12 rice and rice products, 5 wheat and wheat products,

5 grains and cereal based products and 7 different popular varieties of cooked rice and rice products were selected. Phytate content was analysed using anion-exchange chromatography whereas mineral contents were analysed using atomic absorption spectrophotometry (AAS). In general, cooked products had lower content of phytate and minerals as compared to raw products. This could be due to the influence of the cooking method on phytate and mineral content in the food. The results of the study showed that although many of the food samples analyzed had high mineral content, the high phytate content may impair the bioavailability of the mineral in the body[263].

Fortification of common staple foods with zinc alone or in combination with other vitamins and minerals has been proposed as an intervention to increase intake of zinc in populations who consume these foods.

THE CONNECTION BETWEEN ZINC DYSREGULATION AND PSYCHIATRIC ILLNESS.

Dysregulation of zinc metabolism has been associated with reduced immunological functioning, stunted tissue regeneration, growth retardation, gastro-intestinal complaints, ocular and sensory disturbances. Zinc insufficiency is also associated with neuropsychiatric manifestations that can present as altered behavior and cognition, learning disability, and depression[264]. Zinc deficiency has been shown to affect depression as well as schizophrenia.

PATHOPHYSIOLOGY OF ZINC IN THE GENESIS OF DEPRESSION

Clinical studies show lower serum zinc levels in patients with major depression[265-68.] Multiple studies demonstrate reduced serum zinc levels in depressed individuals compared to healthy controls were at least 1.85 μmol/L lower in depressed subjects than control subjects[268]. Zinc supplementation also improved mood in cases with treatment-resistant depression in several studies[267]. Recent meta-analyses demonstrated significant inverse associations between depression severity scores and serum zinc levels and also demonstrated larger effect sizes in hospitalized patients[268]. There exists a correlation between zinc dysregulation in both neurological and psychiatric illnesses such as Parkinson's disease, Alzheimer's, amyotrophic lateral sclerosis, attention deficit disorder hyperactivity and major depression[269]. Consistent with effects and causality, an inverse relationship has been observed between lower zinc levels and higher Hamilton Depression Rating Scale scores[270]. Several randomized controlled trials support the effectiveness of zinc as adjunctive therapy for improving mood in both depressed and healthy individuals[267,271-274]. Clinical studies have shown that low levels of zinc intake contributes to the symptoms similar to depression and patients suffering from depression have a lower serum zinc level[275]. Interestingly, it has been noted that a zinc deficient diet influences the severity of depressive symptoms in women but not in men[276].

1) **DECREASED NEUROGENESIS IN ZINC DEFICIENCY**

It is not well understood how zinc effects its antidepressant activity however these are a few possible ways. Depression is characterized by decreased neurogenesis and enhanced neurodegeneration which, in part, may be caused by inflammatory processes. There is evidence indicating that in depression neurodegenerative processes could be related to dysfunctions affecting the zinc ion availability[277]. It is well-known that zinc deficiency leads to neuronal death in the brain[278].

a) BDNF levels are low in depressive illnesses. Zinc deficiency leads to low BDNF levels and BDNF deficiency in turn decreases neurogenesis and this may predispose to depression[255,279]. An inverse correlation has been observed between serum BDNF levels and severity of depression in a clinical trial[271]. Rodents fed a diet deficient in zinc demonstrated reduced zinc levels in the hippocampal vesicles, an area of the brain that normally has higher concentrations of zinc, with an associated decrease in progenitor cells and immature neurons[255].

b) TrkB is also known as tyrosine receptor kinase B. TrkB is a receptor for brain- BDNF. It was always thought that TrkB receptors were activated in a BDNF-dependent manner. However Huang et al showed that zinc cations released in the CA3 area of the hippocampus not only transactivates TrkB independent of BDNF but that the transactivation produces hippocampal mossy fiber potentiation[280]. Long-term potentiation (LTP) is a persistent strengthening of synapses based on recent patterns of activity. These are patterns of synaptic activity that produce a long-lasting increase in signal transmission between two neurons. LTP is widely considered one of the major cellular mechanisms that form the basis of learning and memory. Further studies with mice suggest that not only zinc is required for mossy fiber potentiation, it can also inhibit it postsynaptically. This suggests that zinc may be required as a dual control to maintain homeostasis[281]. Postpartum mice were fed a zinc-deficient (0.85 ppm) diet and their offspring were used as a lactational zinc deficiency mouse models. Lactational zinc deficiency resulted in lower levels of p-TrkB, in the hippocampus, suggesting that zinc deficiency-induced low levels of TrkB phosphorylation leading to hippocampal neuronal apoptosis. Zinc thus is seen to be playing a role in synaptic plasticity, maintaining neurogenesis and preventing pathological depressive states.

b) **ZINC DIRECTLY INHIBITS NMDA-SENSITIVE GLUTAMATE-GATED CHANNELS**

In the limbic system, zinc accumulates predominantly within glutamatergic neurons, acting as an inhibitory modulator at the NMDA glutamate receptor[282]. Zinc accumulates in the synaptic vesicles of glutamatergic forebrain neurons and modulates neuronal excitability and synaptic plasticity by multiple poorly understood mechanisms. Zinc directly inhibits NMDA-sensitive glutamate-gated channels by two separate mechanisms. Firstly through high-affinity binding to N-terminal domains of GluN2A subunits reducing the channel open probability, then through low-affinity voltage-dependent binding to pore-lining residues blocking the channel.

Antidepressant therapy can increase zinc concentrations in the brain. In the hippocampus, prolonged treatment with antidepressant drugs either imipramine or citalopram increased the ratio of zinc concentrations in the hippocampus/brain regions[282]. In contrast, electroconvulsive therapy, robustly increased zinc concentration in the hippocampus with only a slight effect in the rest of brain. In the cerebral cortex, chronic antidepressant treatment "down-regulated" the density and affinity of the cortical but not hippocampal NMDA receptors. Chronic imipramine treatment increased the ability of zinc ion to inhibit the NMDA receptor complex in the cerebral cortex but not in the hippocampus. Data indicate a complex role of the interaction between zinc and NMDA receptor complex in the mechanism of antidepressant treatment and strongly support the glutamate hypothesis of the mechanism of antidepressant action[282]. A lack of normalization of the zinc level after a course of antidepressant treatment has been suggested to be a marker of drug resistance[283].

c) **INHIBITORY ACTIONS AT GLYCOGEN SYNTHASE KINASE 3 BETA**

Zinc exerts inhibitory actions at glycogen synthase kinase 3beta (GSK3β) which is also pertinent to mechanisms of depression[284]. Abnormal regulation and expression of GSK3β has been associated with an increased susceptibility towards bipolar disorder and other diseases.[285] In the central nervous system, zinc modulates predominantly the excitatory amino acid (glutamatergic) neurotransmission. Glycogen synthase kinase 3 exist in 3 forms namely GSK-3α, GSK-3β and GSK-3β2 and has a major role in Wnt and Hedgehog signaling pathways and regulates the cell-cycle, stem-cell renewal and differentiation, apoptosis, circadian rhythm, transcription and insulin. A large amount of evidence supports the theory that pharmacological inhibitors of GSK-3 may be utilized to treat several diseases, including Alzheimer's disease and other neurodegenerative diseases, bipolar affective disorder and lastly diabetes mellitus \where GSK-3β inhibitors can increase insulin sensitivity,[285].

d) DECREASED ROS GENERATION THROUGH ACTIVATION OF SUPEROXIDE DISMUTASE.

Zinc activates superoxide dismutase (SOD) which is an enzyme that is also an antioxidant as it can catalyzes the dismutation of the superoxide radical into ordinary molecular oxygen and hydrogen peroxide and this decreases reactive oxidation species (ROS).

This process protects the cell. The other major enzymes directly involved in the detoxification of ROS are catalase and glutathione peroxidases. Catalase catalyzes the decomposition of hydrogen peroxide to water and oxygen. Glutathione peroxidases reduce lipid hydro peroxides to their corresponding alcohols. Several subtypes of glutathione peroxidase are selenium dependent. Selenium is a trace mineral that can be taken as a supplement as well.

PATHOPHYSIOLOGY OF ZINC IN THE GENESIS OF SCHIZOPHRENIA

Marger et al reviewed the role of zinc in the central nervous system and discussed the relevance of the most recent association between the zinc transporter (ZIP) 8 and schizophrenia. An enhanced understanding of zinc transporters in the context of ion channel modulation may offer new avenues in identifying novel therapeutic entities that target neurological disorders[259]. Low concentrations of zinc modulate the activity of a multitude of voltage- or ligand-gated ion channels, indicating that this divalent cation must be taken into account in the analysis of the pathophysiology of CNS disorders including epilepsy, schizophrenia and Alzheimer's disease[259].

The role of zinc homeostasis in various psychopathologies is an area of recent interest[286]. How zinc plays a role in depression is rather well illuminated but this is not the case for schizophrenia. There is growing evidence of abnormal zinc transporters associated with schizophrenia[286]. Lower zinc levels in those with schizophrenia may be a consequence of inflammation, genetic defects in molecules that maintain zinc homeostasis, deficient nutritional deficiencies or malabsorption. This can produce NMDA hyperactivity and possibly psychotic symptomatology.

A meta-analysis of serum zinc concentrations in patients with schizophrenia was conducted. This meta-analysis revealed a disturbance of zinc homeostasis in patients with schizophrenia compared to healthy controls, although the relationship between reduced serum zinc levels and psychotic symptoms remains not well explained. Altered serum zinc might be linked to defective transporters and or inflammation that effects the brain's glutamatergic system[286].

A few studies have looked at levels of trace minerals in schizophrenic patients and here is the result. Thirty-nine studies with a total of 5151 participants were included in a meta-analysis of combined plasma and serum data on schizophrenic patients. This meta-analysis revealed an excess of copper, along with deficiencies of zinc, iron, and manganese, in patients with schizophrenia[287]. In a study by Liu et al on 114 schizophrenia patients and 114 healthy controls noted that copper ≤0.97 µg/mL (normal reference range 0.75 to 1.45 µg/ mL) selenium ≤72 ng/mL (normal reference range 70 to 150 ng/mL) and elevated manganese >3.95 ng/mL (normal reference range 1.69 ± 0.40 ng/mL) were associated with an increased risk of schizophrenia[288]. Lower concentrations of copper, selenium iron, arsenic, nickel and aluminum, as well as higher concentrations of manganese and chromium were associated with a more chance of schizophrenia. Yanik et al studied trace elements in patients with a DSM-IV diagnosis of schizophrenia and compared them with sex- and age-matched healthy population[289]. Plasma copper concentrations were significantly higher ($p < 0.01$) and manganese and iron concentrations were lower ($p < 0.05$ and $p < 0.05$, respectively) in schizophrenic patients than in normal population. However unlike previous studies[287,288], selenium and zinc concentrations did not differ between patients and healthy controls. Copper-containing enzymes, include dopamine-beta-hydroxylase and tyrosine hydroxylase, which are linked to the production of dopamine and norepinephrine, which have been involved in the genesis of schizophrenia[288]. Hence malfunctions linked to any of these enzymes due to low copper might be associated with the pathogenesis and etiology of schizophrenia. As far back as 1975, serum copper concentrations were found to be significantly higher in the schizophrenic patients than in the normal control subjects. The average serum copper in schizophrenic females was higher than in schizophrenic males, but the difference was not statistically significant[290]. Levels of certain nutritional essential trace metals iron and selenium were reduced while levels of certain heavy metals lead, chromium and cadmium were raised in schizophrenic patients[291]. **Findings from trace element levels in schizophrenia show a variety of results that are difficult to interpret**[289].

Deficiencies of essential nutrients like amino acids, vitamins, lipids, and trace elements during gestation and early infanthood have potent adverse effects on the development of the limbic system. These effects may be irreversible, even when adequate supplementation is provided at later developmental stages. Recent advances in the neurochemistry of biometals are increasingly establishing the roles of the trace elements iron, copper, zinc, and selenium in a variety of cell functions and are providing insight into the manifestations of deficiencies and excesses of these elements on the development of the central nervous system.[292]

A study by Motzavi et al conducted a study on 30 inpatients with schizophrenia. Patients were randomly allocated into two groups; one group of patients receiving risperidone 6 mg/day as well as zinc sulfate (containing 50 mg elemental zinc) three times a day and another group received risperidone 6 mg/day together with placebo. The Positive and Negative Syndrome Scale (PANSS) was used to assess the psychotic symptoms and aggression risk at baseline, week 2, 4, and 6 of the study. Both groups of treatment modalities significantly decreased scores on every subscale of the PANSS. However, improvement was significantly higher in zinc sulfate receiving group compared to the group receiving placebo. No major clinical side-effects were detected.[293]. This suggest that zinc may have some role to play in the treatment of schizophrenia.

Chapter 14

COGNITION AS A FUNCTION OF THE BRAIN

Cognition is a psychological function of the brain and is an umbrella term for many of its aspects. These are listed below:

1) Being aware of one's surroundings is a function of cognition.
2) Memory can be subdivided into working memory, short term memory and long term memory, visual and auditory memory.
3) Paying attention and concentrating.
4) Planning, organizing, sequencing and abstraction is termed executive function.
5) Reasoning logically and solving problems.
6) Ability to learn new things.
7) Language production.
8) Visual and auditory processing.

1) AWARENESS

The function of being aware is brought about by the reticular activating system (RAS). During sleep we are unaware of our surrounding as the RAS is depressed. This is situated in the brainstem.

2) MEMORY

Working Memory

Working memory is a type of short term memory that has limited capacity. This type of memory is required for executive function. The information held in this type of memory is manipulated while performing tasks or during reasoning. Working memory entails functions such as guarding against external distraction also known as distractor resistance. Distractor resistance entails the prevention of external stimuli from interfering into working memory. In addition it involves the shifting of attention within working memory and collecting new information are other components of working memory[294].

Short term memory

Short- term memory is the transient storing of information in the absence of more information and is essential in enabling advanced cognition[294].

Long term memory

Long-term memory is again divided into two types[295]. Explicit otherwise known as declarative memory and implicit or procedural memory. Declarative memory/ explicit memory means memories that can be are recalled voluntarily[295]. Declarative memory can be further divided into two areas namely episodic memory which pertains to events and experiences and semantic memory which pertains to facts and concepts[295]. Procedural memory or implicit memory is associated with a memory of skills on how to perform skills and it may be executed without being conscious of the action, such as tying a shoelace, playing a violin or riding a bicycle. These memories are typically brought about by repetition and much practice, and consists of automatic sensorimotor behaviors that are well imprinted in our minds[295].

These procedural memories enable the carrying out of various ordinary motor actions in an automatic manner. Acquired skills like driving are kept in the putamen, behavior pertaining to grooming are stored in the caudate nucleus while coordination of body skills involve the cerebellum. Without the medial temporal lobe, a person may still continue to make new procedural memories but will be unable to remember the other events during which it happened[295].

3) **ATTENTION AND CONCENTRATION**

Attention means the ability to maintain the focus[296]. In the reticular activating system, the thalamus has an important role in shifting the focus of attention[296]. The thalami and cerebral cortex receive incoming sensory signals, evaluate the contents, and send out brain resources to execute the requests made. The thalami obtains the information that comes to our senses, then it will relay it to the proper areas of the brain. Concentration is known as the ability to shift that focus from topic to topic[296].

4) **EXECUTIVE FUNCTION**

Executive function refers to planning, organizing sequencing of events and abstract thinking. Executive function takes part in the prefrontal cortex of the brain. It appears to decline during the onset of dementia and hence the person has problem managing his/her own life[296].

5) **REASONING LOGICALLY, JUDGEMENT AND SOLVING PROBLEMS**

Judgement is the ability to reason, problem solve and come to a decision or conclusion.

6) LEARNING

Learning is the ability of humans to understand, remember and use new information, or modify and enhance, existing knowledge, behaviors and skills. Learning involves integrating skills and various aspects of knowledge. The act of learning is a learning curve and happens gradually. Learning builds on itself and accumulates on past knowledge. Learning occurs in many ways, as part of formal education, training and even through personal experience or experience of others. Observational learning was described by Albert Bandura[297] and as the name implies the learning occurs through observation. Learning may also occur as a result of classical conditioning and sometimes it is propelled by motivation

7) LANGUAGE PRODUCTION

There are multiple phases in language production. The message itself is formulated in the thoughts, process of encoding the message into the linguistic form, then encoding the linguistic form into speech, then the audible sound travels from the speaker's mouth to the hearer's ear and to the auditory system in the brain. Speech is decoded into linguistic form and finally the linguistic sound is converted into meaning[298].

8) VISUAL AND AUDITORY PROCESSING

Auditory and visual processing by the brain are required to convert visual and auditory stimuli into meaning in the brain. Any dysfunction here will lead to problems in auditory and visual processing. Individuals with auditory processing disorder cannot make any meaning of the information they hear in the same way as other people do and this causes difficulties in recognizing and understanding speech.

AREAS OF THE BRAIN INVOLVED WITH COGNITION

a) Dorsolateral Prefrontal Cortex

The prefrontal cortex (pfc) is that part area of the brain that deals with executive function. It can be found at the front one third of the brain, beneath the forehead. It is often segregated into three sections:

1) Dorsal lateral section (on the external surface of the pfc),
2) Inferior orbital section (on the anterior undersurface of the brain).
3) Cingulate gyrus (this runs through the middle of the frontal lobes). Cingulate gyrus, is also considered as part of limbic system. The dorsal lateral and inferior orbital gyrus are often termed as the executive control center of the brain.

The functions of prefrontal cortex are listed as -attention, concentration, perseverance, planning, organizing, judgment as well as impulse control. In addition, self-monitoring and supervision, problem solving, critical thinking, forward thinking, learning from experience and mistakes, ability to feel and express emotions influences the limbic system, empathy and lastly internal supervision.

b) Hippocampus

The hippocampus is a tiny part of the brain that is shaped like a sea horse and forms part of the limbic system. The limbic system is situated in the medial temporal lobe towards the center of the brain. The other parts of the limbic system consists of mamillary bodies and amygdala. The hippocampus is associated with long term memory focussing on declarative memory[295] as well as spatial navigation. Declarative memory is a type of memory that is concerned with knowledge, facts and concepts. The hippocampus is not involved with short term memory.

Short term memory is managed by the cerebellum which is located posteriorly as is procedural memory

c) **Basal Ganglia**

A collection of nuclei known as the basal ganglia are found on both sides of the thalamus deep within the cerebral hemispheres. The neurotransmitters at the basal ganglia are gamma amino butyric acid (GABA) and glutamate. The corpus striatum consists of the caudate nucleus, the putamen. The caudate begins from behind the frontal lobe and arches back towards the occipital lobe. It sends information to both frontal lobes. The putamen another basal ganglia structure is situated under and behind the caudate nucleus. The putamen is involved in coordinating automatic behaviours such as bicycle riding and driving. The putamen and caudate play a big part in procedural memory[295].

The globus pallidus is located inner to the putamen, and has two parts, outer part and inner part. It receives inputs from the caudate and putamen and provides outputs to the substantia nigra below. The nigrostriatal pathway is a bilateral dopaminergic pathway in the brain that connects the substantia nigra in the midbrain with the the caudate nucleus and putamen in the forebrain. The substantia niagra is situated at the upper portion of the midbrain and below the thalamus, it is black due to deposition of the pigment neuromelanin.

The nucleus accumbens is situated inferior to the globus pallidus. It receives signals from the prefrontal cortex through the ventral tegmental area and sends other signals back there through the globus pallidus. The basal ganglia are most often linked to the initiation and execution of movements. The basal ganglia is thought to act to facilitate desired movements and inhibit unwanted movements[299.]

d) **Cerebellum**

The cerebellum is located posteriorly. The cerebellum appears like an extra structure attached to the base of the brain. It fits neatly underneath the cerebral hemispheres. Its exterior is covered with finely spaced grooves different from the broad convolutions found in the cerebral cortex. The external surface of the cerebellum resembles an accordian.

It is involved in cognitive operations especially procedural memory as well as short term memory[295]. In addition other operations like attention and language, and in regulating fear and pleasure responses are also cerebellar functions. However its motor functions are well established. While the cerebellum does not initiate movement, it helps in coordination, precision, and accurate timing. It receives information from sensory systems of the spinal cord and from various parts of the brain, and integrates these information to delicate motor functions. Damage to cerebellum produces disorders in fine movement, balance, posture, and motor learning.

e) **Reticular activating system**

The reticular activating system consists of loosely related neurons that are located at the brainstem that project in to the cortex through the thalamus. It functions to switch a person's conscious state from relaxed to highly attentive. It has ascending fibres known as ARAS or ascending reticular activating system[295].

f) **Thalamaus**

The thalamus is a small structure that is located above the brainstem and below the cerebral cortex. The thalamus checks in-comming information with regard to sensation, and ascertains which is most important, and allows only the information which it considers most important to access to higher brain levels[295].

Chapter 15

OVERVIEW OF MAJOR DEPRESSIVE DISORDER

Depression is a psychiatric disorder that was initially described by Hippocrates, and was termed melancholia that meant excess of "Black Bile"[300]. In fact, melancholia is derived from the Greek words, "Melas" meaning black, and "Chole" meaning bile. Our understanding of depression has expanded by leaps and bounds, from Avicenna the 9th century Persian physician describing mood disorders, to Emil Krapelin describing different melancholia as depressive states, and Sir Henry Maudsley, the British psychiatrist who first proposed the overlapping category of affective disorders. New areas of interest around the study of depression are constantly evolving and in this book we relook at nutrition to uncover any roles that supplements may play.

1. EPIDEMIOLOGY

According to the World Health Organization, there are around 4.4% of the total world population or 322 million people in the world currently suffering from depression. It is slightly more common in females (5.1%) compared to males (3.6%), and is more prevalent in older adulthood (age 55-74 years)[301].

2. PATHOPHYSIOLOGY

A) Genetics

There is strong evidence for genetic factors in the development of depressive disorders backed by family and twin studies. Twin studies have shown a heritability of 37%, with family studies showing a double or triple increased risk of developing depression in first degree offspring of patients with depression[302].

Most recent studies:

- CONVERGE study on Chinese women has found associations between 2 single nucleotide polymorphisms on Chromosome 10, one near the *SIRT*-1 gene and another in the intron of LHPP[303]. The importance of this finding lies in the fact that all the participants were Han Chinese women with severe, recurrent depression and this reduced the phenotypic heterogeneity.
- A recent meta analyses shows that there are 102 independent genetic associations with depression[304].

B) Environment and Psychological Stress

Environmental and psychological stress is seen to contribute to the development of depression as well.

a) Childhood stress such as childhood abuse, neglect and loss are known to contribute to depression in later life[305].
b) Life time and recent stress events, sexual abuse, low educational background and childhood trauma were all found to be strongly associated with depression[306].
c) in urban areas, being unemployed, and ironically, being highly paid was associated with higher rates of depression[307]

Interestingly, there is evidence how genetics, interacting with environmental and psychological stress can contribute to the development of depression.

i. The levels of SERT mRNA expression is lower in those with the serotonin transporter (SERT) gene-linked polymorphic region (5-HTTLPR) and prenatal stress and childhood maltreatment. This change in SERT expression is hypothesized to be alter serotonergic functioning and increase the vulnerability to depression[308].
ii. Another study, which explored the associations between gender and 5-HTTLPR, found that while boys carrying the 5- HTTLPR polymorphism were affected by living in public housing rather than privately owned homes, and by living with separated parents. However, in girls, it was found that carrying the 5-HTTLPR polymorphisms were affected by traumatic conflicts within the family[309].
iii. The FKBP5 gene, which has been implicated in the stress-response system, was found to be associated with higher rates of sociodemographic stressors as well as having depression in adolescents[310].

C) Biological and Molecular Mechanisms of Depression

While the molecular mechanisms of depression are still incompletely understood, there is some are a few theories with strong evidence for the biological basis of depression

1) The classical monoamine theory
    The first generation antidepressants (TCAs and MAOIs) cause an increase in the monoamine synaptic concentrations and there is further evidence that there is a deficiency of noradrenaline, serotonin and dopamine in the monoaminergic synapses of individuals with depression[311]. This theory was further expanded to include downregulation and desensitization

of the pre- and post- synaptic noradrenaline and serotonin receptors, as it could better explain the delayed response of antidepressants[312].

2) The hypothalamo-pituitary-adrenal axis (HPA axis)

The HPA axis is activated by stress, hence it has been seen in depressed patients, that there are increased levels of cortisol in the bodily fluids, increased levels of cortisol releasing factor (CRF) in the cerebrospinal fluid and the limbic areas of the brain and increased size and activity of the adrenal and pituitary glands[313]. This is hypothesized to be due to alterations in the feedback inhibition, as evidenced by the absence of cortisol suppression in depressed patients when administered the dexamethasone suppression test[314].

3) Depression and Inflammatory Processes

There is an increase of inflammatory cytokines such as interleukins and tumour necrosis factor alpha (TNF-α) in depressed patients[315]. This is thought to affect the HPA axis as well as the metabolism of the monoamine neurotransmitters[316]. Furthermore, there is evidence T-cell response and activation is also affected in depression, as there is decrease in T-cell response[317].

3. CLINICAL FEATURES

According to the DSM-V[318], the features of Major Depressive Disorder are:-

i. Depressed mood, can appear as irritable in children and adolescents
ii. Reduced interest in activities
iii. Significant weight loss, or a marked change in one's appetite, can be increased or decreased

iv. Difficulty sleeping, or sleeping excessively
v. Appearing increasingly restless, anxious or appearing extremely slow
vi. Feeling extremely tired or having no decreased energy
vii. Feelings of worthlessness or guilt
viii. An inability to concentrate, or finding it difficult to think clearly
ix. Thoughts of death or suicide

CHAPTER 16

OVERVIEW OF BIPOLAR DISORDER

Bipolar Mood Disorder (BMD) (Type 1 and 2) was first conceptualized in the late 19th century, where Jules Baillarger and Jean Pierre Falret independently presented papers describing this illness. While Baillarger called it "Folie a double forme (dual form insanity)", Falret called it "folie circulaire (circular insanity)", and was deemed to be incurable, with a poor prognosis[319]. In modern times, BMD has been brought into the media spotlight, with celebrities such as Demi Lovato, Stephen Fry, and Catherine Zeta-Jones disclosing their struggles with the illness[320]. However, this illness is sometimes poorly understood and our knowledge regarding BMD is constantly evolving, enhancing our insight into this dreaded, and sometimes dramatic illness.

1. EPIDEMIOLOGY

BMD has a lifetime prevalence of around 1%, with Bipolar Mood Disorder Type 1 having a prevalence of 0.6%, and Type 2 having a prevalence of 0.4%[321]. While the onset of illness is usually in the early 20s, a bimodal distribution has also been observed, with one peak in between the ages of 15 and 24, and another peak between the ages of 45 and 54[322] There were no observed differences in the prevalence between sexes or race.

2. PATHOPHYSIOLOGY

A) Genetics

Family and twin studies have shown a strong genetic risk for bipolar mood disorder [323]. The risk in first degree relatives are estimated to be around 9%, which is almost 9 times higher when compared to the general population (1%)[324]. Bipolar Mood Disorder is estimated to be around 85%, which is much higher than most medical disorders, and more than 70% of this heritability is exclusive to the manic syndrome, rather than overlap with major depressive disorder[325].

Polymorphisms in genes of Brain-derived Neurotropic Factor (BDNF), Dopamine Receptor D4 (DRD4), d-amino acid oxidase(DAOA) and Tryptophan Hydroxlase (TPH1) have been found to be significant in certain studies, however when meta analyses was done this was found to be not significant[326]. Hence, the most reliable association were derived from Genome Wide Association Studies (GWAS). Among the genes to be implicated by GWAS include[327]:-

- ANK3, situated on chromosome 10q21.2, which encodes ankyrin B, a protein that is involved in the axonal myelination
- CACNA1C, situated on chromosome 12p13, which encodes for a voltage gated ion channel, playing a role in neuronal development
- TRANK1, situated on chromosome 3p22, encodes a protein which is highly expressed in tissues of the brain

B) Environmental and Psychological Stress

It has been found that life events, more specifically, negative life events can trigger the first episode, as well as subsequent episodes of mania or depression in BMD[328]. Furthermore, according to the "Kindling" theory by Post, earlier episodes in BMD are more likely to be triggered by psychosocial stress, when compared to later episodes[329].

Other environmental factors that have been associated with BMD include maternal smoking[330], climate[331], and childhood trauma[332].

B) Biological and Molecular Mechanisms of Bipolar Mood Disorder

There have been a few theories regarding the clinical manifestations and pathophysiology of BMD. Among them are: -

1) Circadian Rhythm Alterations

    There is a marked difference in levels of melatonin and cortisol in BMD patients resulting in a disruption of the rhythm, and can be seen in all phases of the illness (manic, euthymic, depressive)[333].

2) Dysregulation of Mitochondrial Energy Production

    There is increase ATP production in mania caused by an increase in oxidative phosphorylation. The increase in oxidative phosphorylation is explained by multiple mechanisms, which include increase in calcium ions, oxidative stress and an increase in inflammatory cytokines[334]

3) Oxidative Stress

    There is a change in C-reactive protein (CRP), interleukin-6 (IL-6), brain derived neurotrophic factor (BDNF), and tumour necrosis factor (TNF)-α in different mood phases of BMD, thus providing evidence for the increase of oxidative stress in BMD[335]. Furthermore, it was found that glutathione levels were lower and more oxidized in patients with BMD, and it correlated with the age of onset[336].

4) GABA

    There have been multiple studies using MRS that have demonstrated that brain glutamate levels are higher in patients with BMD, especially in the frontal areas of the brain[337]

3. CLINICAL FEATURES

According to the DSM V,

Bipolar Type 1: - Must have a period of mania. A manic episode is as follows

I. Period of elevated or irritable mood, and increase in goal directed activity or energy, lasting at least 1 week
II. 3 or more of the following

   a. Inflated self esteem
   b. Decreased need for sleep
   c. Increased talkativeness
   d. Flight of ideas
   e. Distractibility
   f. Increase in goal directed activity
   g. Increase in risk taking behavior

III. Severe symptoms causing impairment in function

- Can present with psychosis

Bipolar Type 2:

- Only presence of hypomanic and major depressive episodes, no manic episodes. Hypomanic episodes are not severe enough to cause a marked deterioration of functioning or result in hospitalizations. There also cannot be presence of any psychotic symptoms.

CHAPTER 17

OVERVIEW OF SCHIZOPHRENIA

Schizophrenia is arguably the most dreaded of psychiatric illnesses, and while the term "Schizophrenia" is slightly more than a century old, it is likely that this illness has plagued mankind throughout the eons. The disturbances caused by the illness has been described in ancient Egyptian texts, the Hindu Vedas, Chinese medicinal texts, Greek and Roman literature[338]. In more modern times, the term "demence precoce" was first used by Morel to describe the illness, which its concept was further described and named by Kraepelin as "demence praecox", before the term "schizophrenia" was introduced by Eugene Bleuler in 1911[339]. The term "schizophrenia" has Greek roots, "schizo" meaning "splitting" and "phrene" meaning "mind describing the splitting of the psyche and the subsequent deterioration of the personality[340].

1. EPIDEMIOLOGY

Schizophrenia has a worldwide prevalence of approximately 1%, with age of onset usually in adolescence, while childhood and late onset are relatively rare[341]. The prevalence of schizophrenia is equal in both sexes, however the age of onset of the illness is later in females and clinical manifestations are less severe, leading to a better in prognosis in females[342]. There has been no difference noted in the prevalence between races generally, however in the United States, African and Latino Americans have a disproportionate higher prevalence of schizophrenia when compared to Euro and Asian Americans[343].

2. PATHOPHYSIOLOGY

A) Genetics

Twin studies done have revealed a concordance rate of 41-65% in monozygotic twins and 0-28% in dizygotic twins with heritability estimates of around 80%[344]. However, it is interesting to note that schizophrenia does not display Mendelian inheritance which has been displayed by multiple segregation analyses, despite its high inheritability[345]. Segregation analyses also failed to rule out the major gene hypothesis, which has resulted in multiple studies exploring the link between genetic susceptibility and schizophrenia.

Genes that have been identified that affect the susceptibility to schizophrenia include catechol-O-methyltransferase (COMT), FK506-binding protein 5 (FKBP5) and brain-derived neurotrophic factor (BDNF). Furthermore, genome-wide association studies (GWAS) have identified multiple genes and loci which have helped develop a better understanding into the mechanisms of the manifestation of the disease. Among the areas of interest identified through GWAS are[346]: -

- Major Histocompatibility Complex (MHC) region which has been replicated in multiple studies in different populations
- Transcription Factor 4 (TCF4), which is involved in CNS maturation
- Neurogranin (NRGN), situated on 11q24.2, which is codes for a protein kinase that binds to calmodulin
- Vaccinia-related Kinase 2 (VRK2), a protein kinase that is abundant in actively replicating cells

B) Environmental and Psychological Risk factors

Multiple environmental factors have been identified as well as debated on as possible risk factors for schizophrenia. Obstetric complications have long been associated with an increased risk for schizophrenia, with complications of pregnancy such as bleeding, preeclampsia, gestational diabetes, low birth weight, decreased fetal head circumference, and fetal hypoxia, among others, all being found to be associated with an increased risk for schizophrenia[347]. It is also important to note that while a more recent meta-analysis found that low birth weight was not associated with increased risk, an unwanted pregnancy was significantly associated with an increased risk of schizophrenia[348].

Another interesting factor that increases risk for schizophrenia is being born and growing up in urban areas, and it is postulated that increased social stress in urban settings is possibly the reason for the difference in prevalence[349]. However it is interesting to note that some research has found this difference is not present in low and middle income countries, suggesting that it is possible that other factors are involved as well, such as racial discrimination and disproportionate socio-economic factors[350]. Childhood trauma has also been postulated to have a causal effect with adult psychosis and schizophrenia[351], but later studies suggest that this is not a consistent finding[352].

Drug use has also been associated with schizophrenia, with increasing evidence pointing to a causal relationship between cannabis use and schizophrenia[353]. However, there is significant genetic overlap, as it was found that individuals with higher genetic risk, were more likely to start and consume cannabis more regularly and in larger quantities[354]. While there is little evidence of a causal effect between other drugs and schizophrenia, amphetamines in particular, are known to precipitate a psychotic episode and increase the intensity of symptoms, thus leading to a poorer prognosis[355].

One of the more interesting and yet highly controversial risk factors is that the prevalence of schizophrenia is seen to be higher in migrants[356]. These findings are replicated in multiple countries such as USA, United Kingdom, Netherlands and Sweden among others.

Furthermore, another interesting finding is that the increased risk of developing schizophrenia is also higher in the second generation of migrants, those that were born in the host country, albeit at lower levels when compared to the first generation. However, the reasons on why this occurs is not clearly understood, as the prevalence in the countries of origin of the immigrants have similar levels of prevalence. While institutionalized racism and discrimination have been suggested as possible causes[357], it is still unclear what causes this increase risk and further study needs to be done in this area.

C) **Neurobiological and Molecular Mechanisms of Schizophrenia**

There are many theories regarding the neurobiological and molecular mechanisms of Schizophrenia. Among the more popular and widely researched mechanisms are:

1) Dopamine Dysfunction

    The dopamine hypothesis first rose when all antipsychotics were found to be dopamine antagonists, with their affinity for d2 blockade closely correlating with their potency[358]. While earlier research points to a dopaminergic excess in the striatal areas causing the positive symptoms of schizophrenia, more recent research indicates that the highest dysfunction occurs in the nigrostriatal area. It is also noted that the dopaminergic excess is present even in the prodromal phase, and could result in irreversibly cortical damage[359]. Furthermore, negative symptoms are explained by a decrease of dopamine in the prefrontal cortex[360].

2) Glutamate Abnormalities

    The glutamate hypothesis arose from the observation that glutamate antagonists such ketamine and phencyclidine can mimic the symptoms of schizophrenia[358]. Furthermore, the use of ketamine and phencyclidine can cause of relapse of psychosis in stabilized patients of schizophrenia.

3) Immune System Abnormalities

There have been multiple studies which show increased levels of inflammatory markers in patients of schizophrenia, even prior to initiation of treatment. Furthermore, levels of inflammatory biomarkers are higher during a period of relapse, and would normalize after stabilization of the illness[361].

4) Oxidative stress

There have been evidence that there is an alteration of oxidative enzymes and nitrous oxide causing inflammation, oligodendrocyte abnormalities and mitochondrial dysfunction, among others, are part of the pathophysiology of schizophrenia[362].

3. CLINICAL FEATURES

The clinical features according to DSM V are:

I. 2 or more of the following for a period of 1 month (at least one must be A, B or C)
   A. Delusions
   B. Hallucinations
   C. Disorganized Speech (Derailment or incoherence)
   D. Grossly disorganized or catatonic behavior
   E. Negative symptoms (i.e: avolition, anhedonia, asociality, poverty of speech, blunted affect)

II. Deterioration of functioning from prior to onset of illness

CHAPTER 18

BIOAVAILABILITY OF VITAMIN D$_3$ AND OMEGA 3 FATTY ACIDS

Food plays a distinctive role in the proper functioning of bodily functions as well as providing energy to fuel human activities[363]. In addition, nutrients in food provides avenue for possible beneficial potential against diseases while adequate nutrition has been identified as a possible modifiable risk factor in mental disorders, with influence on the onset and outcome of mental health[82,363-365].

VITAMIN D

Vitamin D is discovered as early as the year 1922, in which its functions on calcium homeostasis and bone health had since been widely discussed[366]. Vitamin D exists in two forms, namely ergocalciferol (vitamin D$_2$) which is found in plants; and cholecalciferol (vitamin D$_3$), which is available in animals[366-368]. Cholecalciferol is also produced endogenously in the skin following exposure of ultraviolet-B light[366,368].

Vitamin D has been linked with cognitive disturbance and psychiatric disorders, including mood disorders and schizophrenia[366]. This includes links on vitamin D deficiency and risk of schizophrenia and depression, as well as general low sun exposure with mood disorders[89,369-371].

BIOAVAILABILITY OF VITAMIN D

Vitamin D absorption is affected by several factors such as molecular forms of vitamin D, dietary lipid and fiber with ingestion of vitamin D, as well as forms of vitamin D upon ingestion[368,372].

Existence of vitamin D in various forms affects its absorption, in which absorption of vitamin D via protein mediated transport depends highly on the affinity of the transporters to different molecular forms of vitamin D[372]. Studies also suggested that 25-hydroxy cholecalciferol $25OHD_3$ and dihydroxy cholecalciferol 1, $25(OH)_2 D_3$ forms were absorbed more efficiently compared to cholecalciferol and ergocalciferol, in which both metabolites' absorption were unaffected by lack of biliary salts[368]. In addition, the hydroxylated $25OHD_3$ form also has better retention compared to the non-hydroxylated forms[368].

Due to its properties as a fat-soluble vitamin, it is hypothesized that lipid stimulates absorption of vitamin D when ingested together in a meal, rendering it to be more bio-accessible[368]. High fiber intake on the other hand, was postulated to reduce bioavailability of vitamin D[373,374].

Bioavailability of vitamin D supplements on the other hand was documented to be high in lactose capsule form, followed by oil form and powder-based form[368,372]. Emulsification and encapsulation are also postulated to improve absorption efficiency of vitamin D supplements rendering it as a research interest of the pharmaceutical industry[368,372].

OMEGA 3 FATTY ACIDS

Lipids play an important role in brain health. Fatty acids are abundantly found in the brain and throughout the central nervous system, playing roles in cell membranes structure, cellular transport, and energy storage[375].

There are many types of fatty acids in human body broadly classified into saturated fatty acids and unsaturated fatty acids[375,376-379]. Unsaturated fatty acids can be further classified into polyunsaturated fatty acids, highly unsaturated fatty acids and monounsaturated fatty acids[82,363,364].

Omega-3 fatty acids are polyunsaturated fatty acids which has been linked with mental health, either from a deficiency of omega-3 fatty acids resulting in mental disorders or successful management of the disorders with α-linolenic acid treatments or supplementations[380-382].

BIOAVAILABILITY OF OMEGA 3 FATTY ACIDS

Bioavailability of omega-3 fatty acids depend on several factors such as chemical form of available fatty acids, whether they are available as triglycerides, phospholipids, ethyl esters or free fatty acids; form of omega-3 ingestion such as in powder form, capsules, tablets, or directly from food; and presence of fat or other nutrients upon ingestion[383-385].

Absorption of omega-3 fatty acids is greater when the fatty acids exist in their free forms (95%), compared to triglycerides (68%) and ethyl esters (20%)[386-389]. In addition, absorption of omega-3 fatty acids is further enhanced by administration via emulsion, usually in the form of fish oil available in commercially[379]. Fat by itself, when ingested together with omega-3 fatty acids, works as emulsifiers and increases absorption of omega-3 fatty acids[114,379]. Calcium on the other hand, forms a complex with free fatty acids when ingested together, leading to decreased availability for absorption[114].

Concise table of RDA and serum levels

	Supplement	Recommended serum levels	RDA
1	Vitamin D3 / calcifediol/ 25 hydroxyvitamin D / 25 (OH) D.	75 nmol/L 30ng/mL *The circulating levels of 25-hydroxyvitamin D or 25 (OH) D are measured when estimating vitamin D_3 levels*[11].	600 IU/d (ages 1–70 years) 800 IU/d (71 years and above)

2	EPA (Omega 3)	There are no known recommended serum levels of EPA for mental illness.	2000 to 3000 mg combined EPA and DHA
3	DHA (Omega 3)	There are no known recommended serum levels of DHA for mental illness	2000 to 3000 mg combined EPA and DHA
4	Magnesium	1.5 to 1.9 m Eq/L 1.7 to 2.2 mg/dL 0.75 to 0.95 mmol/L. *Serum magnesium levels reflect only <1 % of the body's magnesium*[221].	420 micrograms/day (Men) 320 micrograms/day (Women)
5	Folate	Adults 2-20 ng/mL, 2-20 µg/L, 4.5-45.3 nmol/L. Children 5-21 ng/mL, 5-21 µg/L 11.3-47.6 nmol/L *Serum folate is almost entirely in the form of N-(5)-methyl tetrahydrofolate*[238].	400 micrograms/day
6	Zinc	80 to 100 µg/dL 12 to 15 µmol/L *Serum or plasma zinc is the best available biomarker of the risk of zinc deficiency in populations*[260].	11 mg (Men) 8 mg (Women)

REFERENCES

1) Institute of Medicine (US) Committee to Review Dietary Reference Intakes for Vitamin D and Calcium; Ross AC, Taylor CL, Yaktine AL, et al., editors. Dietary Reference Intakes for Calcium and Vitamin D. Washington (DC): National Academies Press (US); 2011. 3, Overview of Vitamin D. Available from: https://www.ncbi.nlm.nih.gov/books/NBK56061/
2) Eyles DW, Smith S, Kinobe R, Hewison M, McGrath JJ. Distribution of the vitamin D receptor and 1 alpha-hydroxylase in human brain. J Chem Neuroanat. 2005; 29: 21–30.
3) Neveu I, Naveilhan P, Menaa C, Wion D, Brachet P, Garabedien M. Synthesis of 1,25-dihydroxyvitamin D3 by rat brain macrophages in vitro. J Neurosci Res. 1994; 38: 214–220.
4) Eyles D, Burne T, McGrath J.Vitamin D in fetal brain development. Seminars in cell and development biology. 2011; 22(6):629-36. doi: 10.1016/j.semcdb.2011.05.004. Epub 2011 Jun
5) Stefanowski B, Antosik-Wójcińska AZ, Święcicki Ł. The effect of vitamin D3 deficiency on the severity of depressive symptoms. Overview of current research. Psychiatr Pol. 2017; 18; 51(3):437-454. doi: 10.12740/PP/66809.
6) Holick MF. The D-lightful vitamin D in child health. Journal of parenteral and enteral nutrition. 2012; 36 suppl. 1, 3012; 9S-19S.
7) Kalueff AV, Eremin KO, Tuohimaa P: Mechanisms of neuroprotective action of vitamin D (3). Biochemistry. 2004; 69:738–741.
8) Losel RM, Falkenstein E, Feuring M, Schultz A, Tillmann HC, Rossol-Haseroth K, Wehling M: Nongenomic steroid action: Controversies, questions, and answers. Physiol Rev. 2003; 83:965–1016.
9) Khoraminya N, Tehrani–Doost M, Jazayeri S, Hosseini A, Djazayery A:Therapeutic effects of vitamin D as adjunctive therapy to fluoxetine in patients with major depressive disorder. Aust N Z J Psychiatry. 2013; 47:271–275.

10) Ross AC, Manson JE, Abrams SA, John F A, Patsy M B, Steven K C, Ramon A DA, J Christopher J G, Richard L G, Glenville J, Christopher S K, Susan T M, Clifford J R, Sue A S. The 2011 report on dietary reference intakes for calcium and vitamin D from the Institute of Medicine: what clinicians need to know. J Clin Endocrinol Metab. 2011; 96(1):53–58.

11) Holick MF, Chen TC. Vitamin D deficiency: a worldwide problem with health consequences. Am J Clin Nutr. 2008; 87 (4):1080S–6S. doi:10.1093/ajcn/87.4.1080S

12) Wyskida M, Wieczorowska-Tobis K, Chudek J. Prevalence and factors promoting the occurrence of vitamin D deficiency in the elderly. Postepy higieny i medycyny doswiadczalnej (Online). 2017; 71198-204.

13) Looker AC, Dawson-Hughes B, Calvo MS, Gunter EW, Sahyoun NR. Serum 25-hydroxyvitamin D status of adolescents and adults in two seasonal subpopulations from NHANES III. Bone. 2002; 30: 771–777.

14) Tangpricha V, Scanlon KS, Chen TC, Holick MF. Vitamin D insufficiency among free-living healthy young adults. Am. J. Med. 2002; 112: 659–662.

15) Hyppönen E, Power C. Hypovitaminosis D in British adults at age 45 y: nationwide cohort study of dietary and life style predictors. Am. J. Clin. Nutr. 2007; 85(3): 860–868.

16) Gannagé-Yared MH, Chemali R, Yaacoub N, Halaby G. Hypovitaminosis D in a sunny country: relation to lifestyle and bone markers. J Bone Miner Res. 2000; 15(9):1856-62 (ISSN: 0884-0431)

17) Quah SW, Abdul Majid H, Al-Sadat N, Yahya A, Su TT, Jalaludin MY. Risk factors of vitamin D deficiency among 15-year-old adolescents participating in the Malaysian Health and Adolescents Longitudinal Research Team Study (MyHeARTs). PLoS ONE. 2018; 13(7): e0200736. https://doi.org/10.1371/journal.pone.0200736

18) Shafinaz IS, Moy FM. Vitamin D level and its association with adiposity among multi-ethnic adults in Kuala Lumpur, Malaysia: a cross sectional study. BMC Public Health. 2016; **16,** 232. https://doi.org/10.1186/s12889-016-2924-1

19) Al-Sadat N, Majid HA, Sim PY, Tin T S, Maznah D, Mohd FAB, Najat D, Saidatul N, Liam M, Marie M C, Muhammad Y J, Vitamin D deficiency in Malaysian adolescents aged 13 years: findings from the Malaysian Health and Adolescents Longitudinal Research Team study (MyHeARTs) BMJ Open 2016;6:e010689. doi: 10.1136/bmjopen-2015-010689

20) Lee DM, Tajar A, Ulubaev A, Pendleton N, O'Neill TW, et al. Association between 25-hydroxyvitamin D levels and cognitive performance in middle-aged and older European men. J Neurol Neurosurg Psychiatry. 2009; 80: 722–729.

21) Wilkins CH, Sheline YI, Roe CM, Birge SJ, Morris JC. Vitamin D deficiency is associated with low mood and worse cognitive performance in older adults. Am J Geriatr. Psychiatry. 2006; 14: 1032–1040.

22) Przybelski RJ, Binkley NC. Is vitamin D important for preserving cognition? A positive correlation of serum 25-hydroxyvitamin D concentration with cognitive function. Arch Biochem Biophys 2007; 15; 460(2):202-5.

23) Chei C L, Raman P, Yin Z X, Shi X M, Zeng Y, Matchar D B. Vitamin D levels and cognition in elderly adults in China. Journal of the American Geriatr. Soc. 2014; 62(11), 2125–29.

24) Llewellyn DJ, Langa KM, Lang IA. Serum 25-hydroxyvitamin D concentration and cognitive impairment. Journal of Geriatric Psychiatry and Neurology. 2009; 22:188–195.

25) Buell JS, Scott TM, Dawson-Hughes B, Dallal GE, Rosenberg IH, Marshall F, Katherine T. Vitamin D is associated with cognitive function in elders receiving home health services. J of Geront. Series A, Biological Sciences and Medical Sciences. 2009; 64:888–95.

26) Laughlin GA, Kritz-Silverstein D, Bergstrom J, Reas ET, Jassal SK, Barrett-Connor E, McEvoy LK. Vitamin D Insufficiency and Cognitive Function Trajectories in Older Adults: The Rancho Bernardo Study. J Alzheimers Dis. 2017; 58(3):871-883. doi: 10.3233/JAD-161295. PMID: 28505973; PMCID: PMC5954988.

27) Soni M, Kos K, Lang IA, Jones K, Melzer D, Llewellyn DJ. Vitamin D and cognitive function. Review Scand J Clin Lab Invest Suppl. 2012; 2 43:79-82. doi: 10.3109/00365513.2012.681969.

28) Darwish H, Zeinoun P, Ghusn H, Khoury B, Tamim H, and Khoury S.Serum 25-hydroxyvitamin D predicts cognitive performance in adults. Neuropsychiatr Dis Treat. 2015; 11:2217–23.

29) Wang Y, Shi Y, Wei H. Calcium Dysregulation in Alzheimer's Disease: A Target for New Drug Development. J Alzheimers Dis Parkinsonism. 2017; 7(5):374. doi: 10.4172/2161-0460.1000374. Epub 2017 Sep 15. PMID: 29214114; PMCID: PMC5713908.

30) Itkin A, Dupres V, Dufrêne YF, Bechinger B, Ruysschaert JM, Raussens V. Calcium ions promote formation of amyloid β-peptide (1–40) oligomers causally implicated in neuronal toxicity of Alzheimer's disease. PloS one. 2011; 6(3)

31) Busche MA, Eichhoff G, Adelsberger H, Abramowski D, Wiederhold KH, Haass C, Staufenbiel M, Konnerth A, Garaschuk O. Clusters of hyperactive neurons near amyloid plaques in a mouse model of Alzheimer's disease. Science. 2008; 19; 321(5896):1686-9.

32) Ganji V, Milone C, Cody MM, McCarty F, Wang YT. Serum vitamin D concentrations are related to depression in young adult US population: the

third national health and nutrition examination survey. Int Arch Med. 2010; 3:29. doi: 10.1186/1755-7682-3-29.

33) May HT, Bair TL, Lappe DL, Anderson JL, Horne BD, Carlquist JF, Muhlestein JB. Association of vitamin D levels with incident depression among a general cardiovascular population. Am Heart J. 2010; 159:6. 1037–1043.

34) Hoang MT, Defina LF, Willis BL, Leonard DS, Weiner MF, Brown ES. Association between low serum 25-hydroxyvitamin D and depression in a large sample of healthy adults: the Cooper Center longitudinal study. Mayo Clin Proc. 2011; 86:11.

35) Kjaergaard M, Joakimsen R, Jorde R. Low serum 25-hydroxyvitamin D levels are associated with depression in an adult Norwegian population. Psychiatry Res. 2011; 190:221–25.

36) Gowda U, Mutowo MP, Smith BJ, Wluka AE, Renzaho AM. Vitamin D supplementation to reduce depression in adults: meta-analysis of randomized controlled trials. Nutrition. 2015; 31:421-29.

37) Spedding S. Vitamin D and depression: a systematic review and meta-analysis comparing studies with and without biological flaws. Nutrients. 2014 Apr 11; 6(4):1501-18. doi: 10.3390/nu6041501. PMID: 24732019; PMCID: PMC4011048.

38) Shaffer JA, Edmondson D, Wasson LT, Falzon L, Homma K, Ezeokoli N, Li P, Davidson KW. Vitamin D supplementation for depressive symptoms: a systematic review and meta-analysis of randomized controlled trials. Psychosom Med. 2014; 76 (3):190-96.

39) Hansen, J.P., Pareek, M., Hvolby, A, Anne S, Tomas T, Eric D, Connie T.Vitamin D3 supplementation and treatment outcomes in patients with depression (D3-vit-dep). BMC Res Notes.2019; 12, 203. https://doi.org/10.1186/s13104-019-4218-z

40) Kjaergaard M, Waterloo K, Wang CE, Almas B, Figenschau Y, Hutchinson MS, Svartberg J, Jorde R: Effect of vitamin D supplement on depression scores in people with low levels of serum 25–hydroxyvitamin D: Nested case–control study and randomised clinical trial. Br J Psychiatry. 2012; 201:360–68.

41) Bracken P, Thomas P, Timimi S, Asen E, Behr G, Beuster C et al. Psychiatry beyond the current paradigm. Brit. J. Psychiat. 2012; 201 (6): 430–34.

42) Stumpf WE, Sar M, Clark SA, DeLuca HF. Brain target sites for 1,25-dihydroxyvitamin D3.Science 1982; 215: 1403–05.

43) Berk M, Sanders KM, Pasco JA, Jacka FN, Williams LJ, Hayles AL, Seetal D. Vitamin D deficiency may play a role in depression. Med. Hypotheses. 2007; 69: 1316–19.

44) Michael J. Berridge. Vitamin D and Depression. Pharmacological Reviews, 2017, 69 (2) 80-92; DOI: https://doi.org/10.1124/pr.116.013227

45) Puchacz E, Stumpf WE, Stachowiak EK, Stachowiak MK. Vitamin D increases expression of the tyrosine hydroxylase gene in adrenal medullary cells. Brain Res. Mol. Brain Res. 1996; 36: 193–96.
46) Garcion E, Sindji L, Leblondel G, Brachet P, Darcy F. 1,25-Dihydroxyvitamin D3 regulates the synthesis of gamma-glutamyl transpeptidase and glutathione levels in rat primary astrocytes.J. Neurochem. 1999; 73: 859–66.
47) Swardfager W, Rosenblat JD, Benlamri M, and McIntyre RS. Mapping inflammation onto mood: Inflammatory mediators of anhedonia. Neurosci Biobehav. 2016; Rev 64:148–66.
48) Wei R and Christakos S. Mechanisms underlying the regulation of innate and adaptive immunity by Vitamin D. Nutrients; 2015. 7:8251–60.
49) Catena-Dell'Osso M, Bellantuono C, Consoli G, Baroni S, Rotella F, and Marazziti D. Inflammatory and neurodegenerative pathways in depression: a new avenue for antidepressant development? Curr Med Chem. 2011; 18:245–55.
50) Leonard B and Maes M. Mechanistic explanations how cell-mediated immune activation, inflammation and oxidative and nitrosative stress pathways and their sequels and concomitants play a role in the pathophysiology of unipolar depression. Neurosci Biobehav. 2012; Rev 36:764–85.
51) Lock JT, Sinkins WG, and Schilling WP. Effect of protein S-glutathionylation on Ca^{2+} homeostasis in cultured aortic endothelial cells. Am J Physiol Heart Circ Physiol. 2011; 300:H493–H506. doi: 10.1152/ajpheart.01073.
52) Blazer DG. Depression in late life: review and commentary. J Gerontol A Biol Sci Med Sci. 2003; 58: 249–65.
53) IOM (Institute of Medicine). Dietary reference intakes for calcium and vitamin D. Washington DC: The National Academies Press; 2011.
54) Lips P. Vitamin D, deficiency and secondary hyperparathyroidism in the elderly: consequences for bone loss and fractures and therapeutic implications. Endocr Rev. 2001; 22:477–501.
55) Hall CA, Reynolds-Iii CF. Late-life depression in the primary care setting: challenges, collaborative care, and prevention. Maturitas. 2014; 79:147–52.
56) Prina AM, Deeg D, Brayne C, Beekman A, Huisman M. The association between depressive symptoms and non-psychiatric hospitalisation in older adults. PLoS One. 2012; 7, e34821.
57) Beaudart C, Buckinx F, Rabenda V, Gillain S, Cavalier E, Slomian J, Jean P, Jean R, Olivier B. The effects of vitamin D on skeletal muscle strength, muscle mass, and muscle power: a systematic review and meta-analysis of randomized controlled trials. J Clin Endocrinol Metab. 2014; 99: 4336–45.
58) Lapid MI, Cha SS, Takahashi PY. Vitamin D and depression in geriatric primary care patients. Clin Interv Aging. 2013; 8:509-14. doi: 10.2147/CIA.S42838. Epub 2013 May 3. PMID: 23667311; PMCID: PMC3650570.

59) Alavi NM, Khademalhoseini S, Vakili Z, Assarian F. Effect of vitamin D supplementation on depression in elderly patients: A randomized clinical trial. Clin Nutr. 2019; 38(5):2065–70. doi:10.1016/j.clnu.2018.09.011
60) Milaneschi Y, Shardell M, Corsi AM, Rosamaria V, Stefania B, Jack M, Luiggi F. Serum 25-hydroxyvitamin D and depressive symptoms in older women and men. J Clin Endocrinol Metab. 2010; 95(7):3225–33. doi:10.1210/jc.2010-0347
61) Robinson M, Whitehouse AJ, Newnham JP, Gorman S, Jacoby P, Holt BJ, Serralha M, Tearne JE, Holt PG, Hart PH, Kusel MM: Low maternal serum vitamin D during pregnancy and the risk for postpartum depression symptoms. Arch Womens Ment Health. 2014; 17:213–19.
62) Aghajafari F, Letourneau N, Mahinpey N, Cosic N, Giesbrecht G. Vitamin D Deficiency and Antenatal and Postpartum Depression: A Systematic Review. Nutrients. 2018; 10(4):478. doi :10.3390/nu10040478
63) Hassan Shaymaa Abd. Indian Journal of Public Health Research & Development. Vitamin D Deficiency and First Trimester Miscarriage A Case Control Study. 2018;9, 12:1645-48.
64) Boerman R, Cohen D, Schulte PF, Nugter A. Prevalence of Vitamin D Deficiency in Adult Outpatients With Bipolar Disorder or Schizophrenia. J Clin Psychopharmacol. 2016; 36(6):588–92. doi:10.1097/JCP.000000000000058
65) Cipriani, A., Saunders, K., Attenburrow, M. Stefaniak J, Panchal P, Stockton S, Lane T, Tunbridge E, Geddes J, Harrison P. A systematic review of calcium channel antagonists in bipolar disorder and some considerations for their future development. Mol Psychiatry. 2016; 21, 1324–32. https://doi.org/10.1038/mp.2016.86
66) Andrade A, Ashton B, Shayna M, Julian B, Juan G, Natalie C, Laura L. "Genetic Associations between Voltage-Gated Calcium Channels and Psychiatric Disorders." International journal of molecular sciences vol. 20, 14 3537. 19 Jul. 2019, doi: 10.3390/ijms20143537
67) Ng F, Hallam K, Lucas N, Berk M. The role of lamotrigine in the management of bipolar disorder. Neuropsychiatr. Dis. Treat. 2007; 3: 463–74.
68) Prabhavalkar KS, Poovanpallil NB, Bhatt LK. Management of bipolar depression with lamotrigine: An antiepileptic mood stabilizer. Front. Pharmacol. 2015; 6:242. doi: 10.3389/fphar.2015.00242.
69) Petrov B, Aldoori A, James C, Kefeng Y, Guillermo P, Lee A, Zhang L, Tao L, Reem A, Jonathan P, Samogyi L, Eugene A, Mary F, Barbara G, Ouliana Z Bipolar disorder in youth is associated with increased levels of vitamin D-binding protein. Transl. Psychiatry.2018; 8, 61. https://doi.org/10.1038/s41398-018-0109-7

70) Delanghe J R, Speeckaert R., Speeckaert, M M. Behind the scenes of vitamin D binding protein: more than vitamin D binding. Best Pract. Res. Clin. Endocrinol. Metab. 2015; 29, 773–786.
71) .Gomme P T & Bertolini J. Therapeutic potential of vitamin D-binding protein. Trends Biotechnol. 2004; 22, 340–45.
72) Trujillo G. & Kew R R. Platelet-derived thrombospondin-1 is necessary for the vitamin D-binding protein (Gc-globulin) to function as a chemotactic cofactor for C5a. J. Immunol. 2004; 173, 4130–36.
73) Kisker O, Shinya O, Christian B, Michal F, Flynn E, Robert A, Bruce Z, Folkman J, Rahul R, Swamy N, Steven S. Vitamin D binding protein-macrophage activating factor (DBP-maf) inhibits angiogenesis and tumor growth in mice. Neoplasia **5**, 2003; 32–40.
74) Yamamoto N. & Homma S. Vitamin D3 binding protein (group-specific component) is a precursor for the macrophage-activating signal factor from lysophosphatidylcholine-treated lymphocytes. Proc. Natl Acad. Sci. USA 1991; 88, 8539–43.
75) Cuomo Alessandro, Maina G, Bolognesi S, Rosso G, Bruno B, Zanobini F, Goracci A, Edvige F, Favaretto E, Irene B, Aruro S, Andrea F. "Prevalence and Correlates of Vitamin D Deficiency in a Sample of 290 Inpatients With Mental Illness." Frontiers in psychiatry. 2019; vol. 10: 167, doi:10.3389/fpsyt.2019.00167.
76) Altunsoy N, Yüksel RN, Cingi Yirun M, Kılıçarslan A, Aydemir Ç. Exploring the relationship between vitamin D and mania: correlations between serum vitamin D levels and disease activity. Nord J Psychiatry. 2018; 72(3):221–25. doi:10.1080/08039488.2018.1424238
77) Naifar M, Maalej Bouali, M Guidara, W Ellouze, A S, Jmal K, Omri S Ayadi, F. Bipolar disorder vulnerability: The vitamin D path. The Canadian Journal of Psychiatry. 2020; 65(3), 184–92. https://doi.org/10.1177/0706743719870513
78) Mitra S, Natarajan R, Ziedonis D, Fan X. Antioxidant and anti-inflammatory nutrient status, supplementation, and mechanisms in patients with schizophrenia. Prog Neuro-Psychopharmacol Biol Psychiatry. 2017; 78: 1–11.
79) Commission S. The abandoned illness: a report from the schizophrenia commission (rethink mental illness, London). 2012.
80) Chowdari KV, Bamne MN, Nimgaonkar VL. Genetic association studies of antioxidant pathway genes and schizophrenia. Antioxid Redox Signal. 2011; 15:2037–45.
81) Rabinowitz J, Levine SZ, Garibaldi G, Bugarski-Kirola D, Berardo CG, Kapur S. Negative symptoms have greater impact on functioning than positive symptoms in schizophrenia: analysis of CATIE data. Schizophr Res. 2012; 137: 147–50.

82) Sarris J, Logan AC, Akbaraly TN, Amminger GP, Balanza-Martinez V, Freeman MP, et al. Nutritional medicine as mainstream in psychiatry. Lancet Psychiatry. 2015; 2: 271–4.
83) Bora E, Akdede BB, Alptekin K. The relationship between cognitive impairment in schizophrenia and metabolic syndrome: a systematic review and meta-analysis. Psychol Med. 2017; 47: 1030–40.
84) Becker A, Eyles DW, McGrath JJ, Grecksch G. Transient prenatal vitamin D deficiency is associated with subtle alterations in learning and memory functions in adult rats. Behavioural Brain Research. 2005; 161(2):306-312. DOI: 10.1016/j.bbr.2005.02.015.
85) Eyles DW, Trzaskowski M, Vinkhuyzen AAE et al. The association between neonatal vitamin D status and risk of schizophrenia. Sci Rep. 2018; 8, 17692. https://doi.org/10.1038/s41598-018-35418-z
86) Mc Grath JJ, Burne TH, Féron F, Mackay-Sim A, Eyles DW. Developmental vitamin D deficiency and risk of schizophrenia: a 10-year update. Schizophr Bull. 2010; 36:1073–78.
87) Samoes B, Silveira C. The role of vitamin D in the pathophysiology of schizophrenia. Neuropsychiatry. 2017; 19;7 (4):362-9.
88) Berger GE, Wood S, Mc Gorry PD. Incipient neurovulnerability and neuroprotection in early psychosis. Psychopharmacology bulletin. 2003; 37(2):79–101.
89) Valipour G, Saneei P, Esmaillzadeh A. Serum vitamin D levels in relation to schizophrenia: a systematic review and meta-analysis of observational studies. J Clin Endocrinol Metab. 2014; 99: 3863–72.
90) Itzhaky D, Amital D, Gorden K, Bogomolni A, Arnson Y, Amital H. Low serum vitamin D concentrations in patients with schizophrenia. Isr Med Assoc J. 2012; 14 (2): 88–92.
91) Crews M, Lally J, Gardner-Sood P, Howes O, Bonaccorso S, Smith S, Murray RM, Di Forti M, Gaughran F. Schizophr Res. 2013; 150(2-3):533-7.
92) Jamilian H, Bagherzadeh K, Nazeri Z, Hassanijirdehi M. Vitamin D, parathyroid hormone, serum calcium and phosphorus in patients with schizophrenia and major depression. Int J Psychiatry Clin Pract. 2013; 17(1):30-4.
93) Berg, A O, Melle I, Torjesen PA, Lien L, Hauf E, Andreassen OA. "A cross-sectional study of vitamin D deficiency among immigrants and Norwegians with psychosis compared to the general population." The Journal of clinical psychiatry 71.12 2010; 1598-1604.
94) Grados D, Salavert J, Ramiro N, Carrion M, Ramirez N, Erra A. AB0890 Is There a Relationship Between Vitamin D and Schizophrenia? Annals of the Rheumatic Diseases 2015; 74:1198.

95) Berg AO, Jørgensen KN, Nerhus M, Athanasiu L, Popejoy AB, Bettella F, et al. (2018) Vitamin D levels, brain volume, and genetic architecture in patients with psychosis. PLoS ONE 13(8): e0200250. doi: 10.1371/journal.pone.0200250. eCollection 2018.
96) Chung Y, Cannon TD. Brain imaging during the transition from psychosis prodrome to schizophrenia. J Nerv Ment Dis. 2015; 203(5):336–41.
97) Hakko H, Jokelainen J, Jones RB, Jarvelin MR, Chant DC, Isohanni M. Vitamin D supplementation during the first year of life and risk of schizophrenia: A finnish birth cohort study. Schizophrenia Research, 2003; Vol: 60, Issue: 1: 44-45.
98) Shivakumar, V, Kalmady S V, Amaresha A C, Jose D, Narayanaswamy J C, Agarwal S M, & ... Gangadhar B N. Serum vitamin D and hippocampal gray matter volume in schizophrenia. Psychiatry Research, 2015; 233(2), 175-79.
99) Cieslak K, Feingold J, Antonius D, Walsh-Messinger J, Dracxler R, Rosedale M, Aujero N, Keefe D, Goetz D, Goetz R, Malaspina D. Low vitamin D levels predict clinical features of schizophrenia. Schizophrenia research. 2014; 1; 159(2-3):543-5.
100) Doğan Bulut, Süheyla B, Dicle G, Berkol T, Eda G, Turker T, Aydemir C."The Relationship between Symptom Severity and Low Vitamin D Levels in Patients with Schizophrenia." PloS one vol. 11,10 e0165284. 27 Oct. 2016, doi:10.1371/journal.pone.0165284
101) Yee JY, See YM, Abdul Rashid NA, Neelamekam S, and Lee J, "Association between serum levels of bioavailable vitamin D and negative symptoms in first-episode psychosis. Psychiatry Res. 2016; 30; 243:390-4.
102) K A Graham KA, Keefe RS, Lieberman JA, Calikoglu AS Lansing KM, and Perkins DO, "Relationship of low vitamin D status with positive, negative and cognitive symptom domains in people with first-episode schizophrenia," Early Intervention in Psychiatry, vol. 9, no. 5, pp. 397–405.
103) Lewis DA. Cortical circuit dysfunction and cognitive deficits in schizophrenia—implications for preemptive interventions. Eur J Neurosci. 2012 Jun; 35(12):1871-8. doi: 10.1111/j.1460-9568.2012.08156.x. PMID: 22708598; PMCID: PMC3383640.
104) Kahn RS, Harvey PD, Davidson M, Keefe RS, Apter S, Neale JM, Mohs RC, Davis KL. Neuropsychological correlates of central monoamine function in chronic schizophrenia: relationship between CSF metabolites and cognitive function. Schizophr Res. 1994; 11(3):217-24.
105) Krivoy A, Onn R, Vilner Y, Hochman E, Weizman S, Paz A, Hess S, Sagy R, Kimhi-Nesher S, Kalter E, Friedman T, Friedman Z, Bormant G, Trommer S, Valevski A, Weizman A. Vitamin D Supplementation in Chronic Schizophrenia Patients Treated with Clozapine: A Randomized, Double-Blind, Placebo-controlled Clinical Trial. EBio Medicine. 2017 Dec; 26:138-145. doi:

10.1016/j.ebiom.2017.11.027. Epub 2017 Dec 2. PMID: 29226809; PMCID: PMC5832639

106) Nerhus M, Berg AO, Kvitland LR, Ingrid D I, Hope S, Sandra R D, Melissa A W, Kristin L R, Ann F, Ole A A, Ingrid M. "Low vitamin D is associated with negative and depressive symptoms in psychotic disorders," Schizophrenia Research. 2016; vol. 178, no. 1-3: 44–49.

107) Ghaderi A, Banafshe H.R., Mirhosseini N et al. Clinical and metabolic response to vitamin D plus probiotic in schizophrenia patients. BMC Psychiatry. 2019; 19: 77.

108) Chiang M, Natarajan R, Fan X. Vitamin D in schizophrenia: a clinical review. Evidence-Based Mental Health 2016; 19:6-9.

109) Yüksel, R. N., Altunsoy, N., Tikir, B., Cingi Külük, M., Unal, K., Goka, S., Aydemir, C., & Goka, E. Correlation between total vitamin D levels and psychotic psychopathology in patients with schizophrenia: therapeutic implications for add-on vitamin D augmentation. Therapeutic advances in psychopharmacology. 2014; 4(6), 268–275.

110) Belvederi Murri M, Respino M, Masotti M, et al. Vitamin D and psychosis: mini meta-analysis. Schizophr Res. 2013; 150(1):235-239. doi:10.1016/j.schres.2013.07.017

111) Sheikhmoonesi, Fatemeh et al. "Effectiveness of Vitamin D Supplement Therapy in Chronic Stable Schizophrenic Male Patients: A Randomized Controlled Trial." Iranian journal of pharmaceutical research. 2016; 15, 4: 941-950.

112) Brown, H.E., Roffman, JL. Vitamin Supplementation in the Treatment of Schizophrenia. CNS Drugs. 2014. 28: 611–622.

113) Cholewski M, Tomczykowa M, Tomczyk M. A Comprehensive Review of Chemistry, Sources and Bioavailability of Omega-3 Fatty Acids. Nutrients. 2018; 4; 10(11):1662. doi: 10.3390/nu10111662. PMID: 30400360; PMCID: PMC6267444.

114) Schuchardt JP, Hahn A. Bioavailability of long-chain omega-3 fatty acids. Prostaglandins Leukot. Essent. Fat. Acids. 2013; 89:1–8. doi: 10.1016/j.plefa.2013.03.010.

115) Chapkin RS, McMurray DN, Davidson LA, Patil BS, Fan YY, Lupton JR: Bioactive dietary long-chain fatty acids: emerging mechanisms of action. Br J Nutr 2008; 100(6): 1152–7.

116) Simopoulos AP: Omega-6/omega-3 essential fatty acids: biological effects. World Rev Nutr Diet 2009; 99: 1–16

117) Perica MM, Delas I. "Essential fatty acids and psychiatric disorders". Nutrition in Clinical Practice.2011; 26 (4): 409–25. doi:10.1177/0884533611411306. PMID 21775637.

118) Montgomery P, Richardson AJ. "Omega-3 fatty acids for bipolar disorder". The Cochrane Database of Systematic Reviews.2008; (2): CD005169. doi:10.1002/14651858.CD005169.pub2. PMID 18425912
119) Ruxton CH, Calder PC, Reed SC, Simpson MJ. "The impact of long-chain n-3 polyunsaturated fatty acids on human health". Nutrition Research Reviews. 2005; 18 (1): 113–29. doi:10.1079/nrr200497. PMID 19079899.
120) Robinson LE, Mazurak VC. "N-3 polyunsaturated fatty acids: relationship to inflammation in healthy adults and adults exhibiting features of metabolic syndrome". Lipids. 2013; 48 (4): 319–32. doi:10.1007/s11745-013-3774-6. PMID 23456976.
121) Ajith TA. A Recent Update on the Effects of Omega-3 Fatty Acids in Alzheimer's Disease. Curr Clin Pharmacol 2018; 13(4):252-260. doi: 10.2174 /1574884713666180807145648.
122) Ng TKW, Nalliah S, Hamid A, Wong SR, Sim Ling Chee, Augustine CA. Omega-6 and omega-3 fatty acid nutrition amongst Malaysians are far from desirableIe JSME 2012 6(2): 4-9.
123) Couëdelo L, Amara S, Lecomte M, Meugnier E, Monteil J, Fonseca L, Pineau G, Cansell M, Carrière F, Michalski MC, Vaysse C. Impact of various emulsifiers on ALA bioavailability and chylomicron synthesis through changes in gastrointestinal lipolysis. Food Funct. 2015; 6:1726–1735. doi: 10.1039/C5FO00070J.
124) Ng TK. Omega 3 Fatty Acids: Potential sources in the Malaysian diet with the goal towards achieving recommended nutrient intakes. Mal. J Nutr. M.2006; 12(2):181-188.
125) Singh, M. Essential fatty acids, DHA and human brain. Indian J Pediatr. 2005; **72,** 239–242. https://doi.org/10.1007/BF02859265
126) U.S. Department of Agriculture, Agricultural Research Service. Nutrient Intakes from Food: Mean Amounts Consumed per Individual, One Day, 2005-2006. Available at http://www.ars.usda.gov/SP2UserFiles/Place/12355000/pdf/0506/Table_1_NIF_05.pdf; accessed March 21, 2014.
127) Superko HR, Superko AR, Lundberg GP, Margolis B, Garrett BC, Nasir K, Agatston AS. Omega-3 Fatty Acid Blood Levels Clinical Significance Update. Curr Cardiovasc Risk Rep. 2014; 8(11):407. doi: 10.1007/s12170-014-0407-4. PMID: 25285179; PMCID: PMC4176556.
128) Institute of Medicine, Food and Nutrition Board. Dietary reference intakes for energy, carbohydrate, fiber, fat, fatty acids, cholesterol, protein, and amino acids (macronutrients). Washington, DC: National Academy Press; 2005.
129) Lo Van, A., Sakayori, N., Hachem, m, Mounir B, Madeline Picq, Baptiste F, Lagarde M, Osumi N, Nathalie B.Targeting the Brain with a Neuroprotective Omega-3 Fatty Acid to Enhance Neurogenesis in Hypoxic Condition in

Culture. Mol Neurobiol **56,** 986–999 (2019). https://doi.org/10.1007/s12035-018-1139-0

130) WHO | Dementia. WHO. World Health Organization; 2016
131) Lourida I, Soni M, Thompson-Coon J, Purandare N, Lang IA, Ukoumunne OC, et al. Mediterranean Diet Cognitive Function and Dementia. Epidemiology 2013; 24:479–489. doi:
132) Morris MC. Nutrition and risk of dementia:overview and methodological issues. Ann N Y Acad Sci. 2017; 1367:31–37. doi:
133) Oulhaj A, Jernerén F, Refsum H, Smith AD, de Jager CA. Omega-3 Fatty Acid Status Enhances the Prevention of Cognitive Decline by B Vitamins in Mild Cognitive Impairment. J Alzheimers Dis. 2016; 50: 547–557. doi:
134) Bauer I, Crewther S, Pipingas A, Sellick L, Crewther D. Does omega-3 fatty acid supplementation enhance neural efficiency? A review of the literature. Human Psychopharmacolgy. 2014; 29, (1).1-103.
135) Bauer I, Hughes M, Rowsell R, Cockerell R, Pipingas A, Crewther S, Crewther D. Omega-3 supplementation improves cognition and modifies brain activation in young adults. Human Psychopharmacology: Clinical and Experimental. 2014 Mar; 29(2):133-44.
136) Zhang J, Hebert JR, Muldoon MF: Dietary fat intake is associated withpsychosocial and cognitive functioning of school-aged children in the United States. J Nutr 2005; 135(8): 1967–73
137) Stonehouse W, Conlon CA, Podd J, Stephen H, Anne M, Crystal H, David K. DHA supplementation improved both memory and reaction time in healthy young adults: a randomized controlled trial. Am J Clin Nutr 2013; 97(5): 1134–43.
138) Cook R L, Parker HM, Donges CE, Nicholas J, Cheng H, Katherine S, Cox E, Janet F, Manohar G, Helen T.Omega-3 polyunsaturated fatty acids status and cognitive function in young women. Lipids Health Dis 18, 194 (2019). https://doi.org/10.1186/s12944-019-1143-z
139) Baleztena J, Ruiz-Canela M, Sayon-Orea C, Pardo M, Añorbe T, Gost JI, Gomez C, Ilarregui B, Bes-Rastrollo M. Association between cognitive function and supplementation with omega-3 PUFAs and other nutrients in ≥ 75 years old patients: A randomized multicenter study. PLoS One. 2018 Mar 26; 13(3):e0193568. doi: 10.1371/journal.pone.0193568. PMID: 29579102; PMCID: PMC5868762.
140) Agostoni C, Zuccotti GV, Radaelli G, et al: Docosahexaenoic acid supplementation and time at achievement of gross motor milestones in healthy infants: a randomized, prospective, double-blind, placebo-controlled trial. Am J Clin Nutr 2009; 89(1): 64–70.

141) Nurk E, Drevon CA, Refsum H, et al: Cognitive performance among the elderly and dietary fish intake: the Hordaland Health Study. Am J Clin Nutr 2007; 86(5): 1470–8.

142) Kalmijn S, van Boxtel MP, Ocke´ M, Verschuren WM, Kromhout D, Launer LJ: Dietary intake of fatty acids and fish in relation to cognitive performance at middle age. Neurology 2004; 62(2): 275–80

143) Fontani G, Corradeschi F, Felici A, Alfatti F, Migliorini S, Lodi L. Cognitive and physiological effects of Omega-3 polyunsaturated fatty acid supplementation in healthy subjects. European journal of clinical investigation. 2005; 35(11):691-9.

144) Jackson PA, Deary ME, Reay JL, Scholey AB, Kennedy DO: No effect of 12 weeks' supplementation with 1 g DHA-rich or EPA-rich fish oil on cognitive function or mood in healthy young adults aged 18-35 years.Br J Nutr 2012; 107(8): 1232–43.

145) van de Rest O, Geleijnse JM, Kok FJ, Staveren WA, Dullemeijer C, Olderikkert C, Beekman A, Groot CP. Effect of fish oil on cognitive performance in older subjects: a randomized, controlled trial. Neurology 2008; 71(6): 430–8

146) Horrobin D, Peet M: A dose-ranging study of ethyl-eicosapentaenoatein treatment-unresponsive depression. Biol Psychiatry 2001; 49: 37S.

147) Frangou S, Lewis M, McCrone P: Efficacy of ethyl-eicosapentaenoicacid in bipolar

148) Sinn N: Nutritional and dietary influences on attention deficit hyperactivity disorder. Nutr Rev 2008; 66(10): 558–68

149) Deacon G, Kettle C, Hayes D, Dennis C. & Tucci, J. Omega 3 polyunsaturated fatty acids and the treatment of depression. Crit. Rev. Food Sci. Nutr. 2017; 57, 212–223.

150) Liao Y, Xie B, Zhang H, He Q, Guo L, Subramaniapillai M, Fan B, Lu C, McIntyre RS. Efficacy of omega-3 PUFAs in depression: A meta-analysis. Transl Psychiatry. 2019 Aug 5; 9(1):190. doi: 10.1038/s41398-019-0515-5. PMID: 31383846; PMCID: PMC6683166.

151) Grosso G, Pajak A, Marventano S, Castellano S, Galvano F, Bucolo C, Drago F, Caraci F. Role of omega-3 fatty acids in the treatment of depressive disorders: a comprehensive meta-analysis of randomized clinical trials. PLoS One. 2014 May 7;9 (5):e96905. doi: 10.1371/journal.pone.0096905. PMID: 24805797; PMCID: PMC4013121.

152) Sublette M. E, Ellis S P, Geant A L & Mann J J. Meta-analysis of the effects of eicosapentaenoic acid (EPA) in clinical trials in depression. J. Clin. Psychiatry. 2011; 72, 1577–1584.

153) Hallahan B, Ryan T, Hibbeln JR, Murray IT, Glynn S, Ramsden CE, et al. Efficacy of omega-3 highly unsaturated fatty acids in the treatment of

depression. British Journal of Psychiatry. [Online] Cambridge University Press; 2016; 209(3): 192–201. Available from: doi:10.1192/bjp.bp.114.160242

154) Peet M. & Horrobin D F. A dose-ranging exploratory study of the effects of ethyl-eicosapentaenoate in patients with persistent schizophrenic symptoms. J. Psychiatr. Res. 2002; 36, 7.

155) Song C, shieh CH, Wu YS, Kalueff A, Gaikwd S, Su PK. The role of omega-3 polyunsaturated fatty acids eicosapentaenoic and docosahexaenoic acids in the treatment of major depression and Alzheimer's disease: acting separately or synergistically? Prog. Lipid Res. 2016; 62, 41–54.

156) Mischoulon D, Best-Popescu C, Michael L, Merens W, Murakami JL; Wu S L, Papakostas GI, Dording, C M; Sonawalla S B, Nierenberg AA; Alpert J E, Fava M. A double-blind dose-finding pilot study of docosahexaenoic acid (DHA) for major depressive disorder. Eur. Neuropsychopharmacol. 2008; 18, 639–645.

157) Mocking RJ, Harmsen I, Assies J, Koeter MW, Ruhé HG, Schene AH. Meta-analysis and meta-regression of omega-3 polyunsaturated fatty acid supplementation for major depressive disorder. Transl Psychiatry. 2016 Mar 15; 6(3):e756. doi: 10.1038/tp.2016.29. PMID: 26978738; PMCID: PMC4872453.

158) Wani A L, Bhat S A & Ara A. Omega-3 fatty acids and the treatment of depression: a review of scientific evidence. Integr. Med. Res. 2015. 4, 132–141.

159) Chen CT, Anthony D, Trepanier M, Zhen L, Masoodi M, Richard B. The low levels of eicosapentaenoic acid in rat brain phospholipids are maintained via multiple redundant mechanisms[S]. J. Lipid Res. 2013; 54, 2410–2422.

160) Członkowska, A. & Kurkowska-Jastrzębska, I. Inflammation and gliosis in neurological diseases-clinical implications. J. Neuroimmunol. 2011. 231, 78–85.

161) Mullen A, Loscher CE, Roche HM. Anti-inflammatory effects of EPA and DHA are dependent upon time and dose-response elements associated with LPS stimulation in THP-1-derived macrophages. J Nutr Biochem. 2010; 21(5):444-450.

162) Frangou S, Lewis M, Wollard J. & Simmons A. Preliminary in vivo evidence of increased N-acetyl-aspartate following eicosapentanoic acid treatment in patients with bipolar disorder. J. Psychopharmacol. 2007; 21, 435–439.

163) Moffett JR, Ross B, Arun P, Madhavarao CN, Namboodiri AM. N-Acetylaspartate in the CNS: from neurodiagnostics to neurobiology. Prog Neurobiol. 2007 Feb;81(2):89-131. doi: 10.1016/j.pneurobio.2006.12.003. Epub 2007 Jan 5. PMID: 17275978; PMCID: PMC1919520.

164) .Wu A, Ying Z & Gomezpinilla F. Dietary omega-3 fatty acids normalize BDNF levels, reduce oxidative damage, and counteract learning disability after traumatic brain injury in rats. J. Neurotrauma. 2004; **21**, 1457–1467.

165) .Rao, M. S., Hattiangady, B. & Shetty, A. K. Fetal hippocampal CA3 cell grafts enriched with FGF-2 and BDNF exhibit robust long-term survival and integration and suppress aberrant mossy fiber sprouting in the injured middle-aged hippocampus. Neurobiol. 2006; **21**, 276–290.
166) Binder DK, Scharfman HE. Brain-derived neurotrophic factor. Growth Factors. 2004 Sep; 22(3):123-31. doi: 10.1080/08977190410001723308. PMID: 15518235; PMCID: PMC2504526.
167) Bathina S, Das UN. Brain-derived neurotrophic factor and its clinical implications. Arch Med Sci. 2015 Dec 10; 11(6):1164-78. doi: 10.5114/aoms.2015.56342. Epub 2015 Dec 11. PMID: 26788077; PMCID: PMC4697050.
168) McNamara RK, Able J, Liu Y, Jandacek R, Rider T, Tso P, Lipton JW. Omega-3 fatty acid deficiency during perinatal development increases serotonin turnover in the prefrontal cortex and decreases midbrain tryptophan hydroxylase-2 expression in adult female rats: dissociation from estrogenic effects. J Psychiatr Res. 2009; 43 (6):656-63. doi: 10.1016/j.jpsychires.2008.09.011. Epub 2008 Nov 4. PMID: 18986658; PMCID: PMC2679262.
169) Chan E J, Cho L. What can we expect from omega-3 fatty acids? Cleve. Clin. J. Med.2009; 76, 245–251.
170) Günther J, Schulte K, Wenzel D, Malinowska B, Schlicker E. Prostaglandins of the E series inhibit monoamine release via EP3 receptors: proof with the competitive EP3 receptor antagonist L-826,266. Naunyn Schmiedebergs Arch. Pharmacol. 2010; 381, 21–31.
171) Schlicker E, Fink K, Göthert M.Influence of eicosanoids on serotonin release in the rat brain: inhibition by prostaglandins E1 and E2. Naunyn Schmiedebergs Arch. Pharmacol. 1987; 335, 646–651.
172) Rees D, Miles E A, Banerjee T, Wells S J, Roynette, C. E., Wahle, K. W., Calder, P. C. Dose-related effects of eicosapentaenoic acid on innate immune function in healthy humans: a comparison of young and older men. Am. J. Clin. Nutr. 2006; 83, 331–342.
173) Vedin I, Cederholm T, Freund-Levi Y, Basun H, Hjorth E., Irving G F, Eriksdotter-Jönhagen, M., Schultzberg, M, Wahlund L O, Palmblad J. Reduced prostaglandin F2 alpha release from blood mononuclear leukocytes after oral supplementation of omega3 fatty acids: the OmegAD study. J. Lipid. 2010;
174) Hibbeln, J R, Linnoila, M, Umhau, J C, Rawlings R., George D T, Salem, N, Jr. Essential fatty acids predict metabolites of serotonin and dopamine in cerebrospinal fluid among healthy control subjects, and early- and late-onset alcoholics. Biol. Psychiatry. 1998; 44, 235–242.

175) Way B M, Laćan, G, Fairbanks L A, Melega, W P. Architectonic distribution of the serotonin transporter within the orbitofrontal cortex of the vervet monkey. Neuroscience. 2007; 148, 937–948

176) Crockett M. J. The neurochemistry of fairness: clarifying the link between serotonin and prosocial behavior. Ann. N. Y. Acad. Sci. 2009; 1167, 76–86.

177) Blair R J. A cognitive developmental approach to mortality: investigating the psychopath. Cognition. 1995; 57, 1–29.

178) Healy-Stoffel M, Levant B. N-3 (Omega-3) Fatty Acids: Effects on Brain Dopamine Systems and Potential Role in the Etiology and Treatment of Neuropsychiatric Disorders. CNS Neurol Disord Drug Targets. 2018; 17(3):216-232. doi: 10.2174/1871527317666180412153612. PMID: 29651972; PMCID: PMC6563911.

179) Rhonda PP, Bruce NA. Vitamin D and the omega-3 fatty acids control serotonin synthesis and action, part 2: relevance for ADHD, bipolar disorder, schizophrenia, and impulsive behavior. FASEB J. 2015 Jun; 29 (6):2207-22. doi: 10.1096/fj.14-268342.

180) Sinn N, Milte C, Howe P R. Oiling the brain: a review of randomized controlled trials of omega-3 fatty acids in psychopathology across the lifespan. Nutrients. 2010; 2, 128–170.

181) Lopez VA, Detera-Wadleigh S, Cardona I, Kassem L, McMahon F J; National Institute of Mental Health Genetics Initiative Bipolar Disorder Consortium. Nested association between genetic variation in tryptophan hydroxylase II, bipolar affective disorder, and suicide attempts. Biol. Psychiatry. 2007; 61, 181–186.

182) Sublette M E, Hibbeln J R, Galfalvy H, Oquendo M A, Mann J J. Omega-3 polyunsaturated essential fatty acid status as a predictor of future suicide risk. Am. J. Psychiatry 2006; 163.

183) Hallahan B, Hibbeln J R, Davis J M., Garland M R. Omega-3 fatty acid supplementation in patients with recurrent self-harm. Single-centre double-blind randomised controlled trial. Br. J. Psychiatry. 2017; 190, 118–122

184) Appleton KM, Fraser W D, Rogers P J, Ness, A R., Tobias, J H. Supplementation with a low-moderate dose of n-3 long-chain PUFA has no short-term effect on bone resorption in human adults. Br. J. Nutr. 2011;105, 1145–1149.

185) Bloch M H, Hannestad J. Omega-3 fatty acids for the treatment of depression: systematic review and meta-analysis. Mol. Psychiatry. 2012; 17, 1272–1282.

186) Martins J G, Bentsen H, Puri B K. Eicosapentaenoic acid appears to be the key omega-3 fatty acid component associated with efficacy in major depressive disorder: a critique of Bloch and Hannestad and updated meta-analysis. Molec. Psychiatry. 2012; 17, 1144–1149.

187) Mischoulon, D. The impact of omega-3 fatty acids on depressive disorders and suicidality: can we reconcile 2 studies with seemingly contradictory results? J. Clin. Psychiatry. 2011; 72, 1574–1576.
188) US Department of Agriculture, ARS. 2014. Nutrient Intakes from Food: Mean Amounts Consumed per Individual, by Gender and Age, US Department of Agriculture, Washington, DC.
189) McNamara RK, Nandagopal JJ, Strakowski SM, DelBello MP. Preventative strategies for early-onset bipolar disorder: Towards a clinical staging model. CNS Drugs. 2010; 24:983–96.
190) Akbar M, Calderon F, Wen Z, and Kim H Y. (2005) Proc. Natl. Acad.Sci. U. S. A., 10 10858–1086319.
191) Calderon, F., and Kim, H. Y. J. Neurochem. 2004; 90,979–988
192) Markiewicz I, and Lukomska B. Acta Neurobiol. 2006; Exp. (Wars.)66,343–358
193) Kim HY. Novel metabolism of docosahexaenoic acid in neural cells. J. Biol. Chem. 2007; 282, 18661—18665.
194) Moore, S A. J. Mol. Neurosci. 2001; 16, 195–200.
195) Noaghiul S, Hibbeln JR. Cross-national comparisons of seafood consumption and rates of bipolar disorders. Am. J. Psychiatry160, 2222–2227 (2003)
196) McNamara RK. Evaluation of docosahexaenoic acid deficiency as a preventable risk factor for recurrent affective disorders: Current status, future directions, and dietary recommendations. Prostaglandins Leukot Essent Fatty Acids. 2009; 8:223–31
197) McNamara R. Long-chain omega-3 fatty acid deficiency in mood disorders: Rationale for treatment and prevention. Curr Drug Discov Technol. 2011; 15: 156–61.
198) Shakeri J, Khanegi M, Golshani S, Farnia V, Tatari F, Alikhani M, Nooripour R, Ghezelbash MS. Effects of Omega-3 Supplement in the Treatment of Patients with Bipolar I Disorder. Int J Prev Med. 2016; 19; 7:77. doi: 10.4103/2008-7802.182734. PMID: 27280013; PMCID: PMC4882968.
199) Youdim KA, Martin A, Joseph JA. Essential fatty acids and the brain: possible health implications. Int. J. Dev. Neurosci. 2000; 18(4/5), 383—399.
200) Balanzá-Martínez V, Fries GR, Colpo GD, Silveira PP, Portella AK, Tabarés-Seisdedos R, et al. Therapeutic use of omega-3 fatty acids in bipolar disorder. Expert Rev Neurother. 2011; 11:1029–47.
201) Safari M, Sadr S, Mirabzadeh K, Saki M. The Effect Of Omega 3 And Fluvoxamine On The Depresive Phase In Bipolar Disorder Type I.
202) van der Gaag M, Smit F, Bechdolf A, French P, Linszen D H, Yung A R, McGorry P, & Cuijpers P. Preventing a first episode of psychosis: meta-analysis of randomized controlled prevention trials of 12month and longer-term follow-ups. Schizophrenia research. 2013; 149(1), 56-62.

203) Fusar-Poli P, and Berger G. Eicosapentaenoic acid interventions in schizophrenia: meta-analysis of randomized, placebo-controlled studies. J Clin Psych. 2012; 32: 179-185.
204) Amminger GP, Schäfer MR, Papageorgiou, Claudia K, Sue M, Susan H, Andrew M, Patrick D, Gergor B. Long-chain omega-3 fatty acids for indicated prevention of psychotic disorders: a randomized, placebo-controlled trial. Arch Gen Psychiatry. 2010; 67:146-154.
205) Amminger G P, Schäfer M R, Schlögelhofer M, Klier CM, & McGorry P D. Longer-term outcome in the prevention of psychotic disorders by the Vienna omega-3 study. Nature communications. 2015; 6. 7934.
206) Mossaheb N, Schloegelhofer M, Schaefer MR, et al. Polyunsaturated fatty acids in emerging psychosis. Curr Pharm Des. 2010; 18: 576-591.
207) Smesny S, Milleit, B, Hipler U, Schäfer MR, Klier CM, Holub H, Holzer I, Berger GE, Otto M, Nenadic I, Berk M, McGorry PD, Sauer H, Amminger GP. Omega-3 fatty acid supplementation changes intracellular phospholipase A_2 activity and membrane fatty acid profiles in individuals at ultra-high risk for psychosis. Mol Psychiatry. 2014; 19, 317–324.
208) Marano G, Traversi G, Nannarelli C, Mazza S, Mazza M. Omega-3 fatty acids and schizophrenia: evidences and recommendations. Clin Ter. 2013; 164(6):e529-37. doi: 10.7417/CT.2013.1651. Review.
209) Sethom M.M., Fares S, Bouaziz N. Polyunsaturated fatty acids deficits are associated with psychotic state and negative symptoms in patients with schizophrenia. Prostaglandins Leukot. Essent. Fat. Acids. 2010; 83:131–136.
210) Satogami K, Takahashi S, Yamada S, Ukai S, Shinosaki K. Omega-3 fatty acids related to cognitive impairment in patients with schizophrenia. Schizophr Res Cogn. 2017; 18;9:8-12. doi: 10.1016/j.scog.2017.05.001. PMID: 28740828; PMCID: PMC5514384.
211) Bos DJ, van Montfort SJ, Oranje B, Durston S, Smeets PA. Effects of omega-3 polyunsaturated fatty acids on human brain morphology and function: what is the evidence? Eur. Neuropsychopharmacol. 2016; 26:546–561.
212) Qiao Y, Mei Y, Han H, Liu F, Yang XM, Shao Y, Xie B. Effects of Omega-3 in the treatment of violent schizophrenia patients. Schizophrenia Research. 2018;195 :283-285.
213) Dyall SC. Long-chain omega-3 fatty acids and the brain: a review of the independent and shared effects of EPA, DPA, and DHA. Front. Aging Neurosci. 2015; 21:7–52.
214) Bentsen H, Solberg DK, Refsum H, Bøhmer T. Clinical and biochemical validation of two endophenotypes of schizophrenia defined by levels of polyunsaturated fatty acids in red blood cells. Prostaglandins Leukot. Essent. Fat. Acids. 2012; 87:35–41.

215) van der Kemp WJ, Klomp DW, Kahn RS, Luijten PR, Hulshoff Pol H.E. A meta-analysis of the polyunsaturated fatty acid composition of erythrocyte membranes in schizophrenia. Schizophr. Res. 2012; 141:153–161.
216) Condray R., Yao JK, Steinhauer SR., van Kammen DP, Reddy R.D, Morrow L.A. Semantic memory in schizophrenia: association with cell membrane essential fatty acids. Schizophr. Res. 2008; 106:13–28.
217) Jeroen H F de Baaij, Joost G J H and René J M B. Magnesium in Man: Implications for Health and Disease. Physiological Reviews. vol. 95, no1.
218) Bairoch A. The enzyme database in 2000. Nucleic Acids Res. 2000; 1; 28(1):304-5. doi: 10.1093/nar/28.1.304. PMID: 10592255; PMCID: PMC102465.
219) Ron C, Tomer A, Kate D, Carol A. F, Pallavi S, Ingrid M. K, Anamika K, Markus K, Mario L, Lukas A M, Quang O, Suzanne P, Anuradha P, Alexander G, Michael T, Deepika W, Peifen Z, Peter D K. The Meta Cyc database of metabolic pathways and enzymes and the Bio Cyc collection of pathway/genome databases, Nucleic Acids Research, Volume 40, Issue D1, 1 January 2012, Pages D742–D753, https://doi.org/10.1093/nar/gkr1014
220) Worthington V. Nutritional quality of organic versus conventional fruits, vegetables and grains. J Altern. Complement Med 2001; 7: 161-173.
221) Hansen B, Bruserud. Hypomagnesemia in critically ill patients. J Intensive Care. 2018; 6, 21. https://doi.org/10.1186/s40560-018-0291-y
222) Ismarulyusda I, Zaleha Md I, Jamaludin M, Khairul O, Iskandar Z A, Khalid A K, Osman A. Micronutrient levels among aborigines in Pahang and Perak. Jabatan Ir'esiltatarz Masyarakat 2005: Jilid 11
223) King DE, Mainous AG, Geesey M.E, Woolson R.F. Dietary magnesium and C-reactive protein levels. J. Am. Coll. Nutr. 2005; 243:166–171.
224) Galan P, Preziosi P, Durlach V, Valeix P, Ribas L, Bouzid D, Favier A, Hercberg S. Dietary magnesium intake in a French adult population. Magnes. Res. 1997; 104:321–328.
225) Institute of medicine us standing committee on the scientific evaluation of dietary reference intakes. Dietary Reference Intake for Calcium, Phosphorous, Magnesium, Vitamin D and Fluoride. Washington, DC National Academic Press, 1997.
226) Jiang P, Lv Q, Lai T, Xu F. Does Hypomagnesemia Impact on the Outcome of Patients Admitted to the Intensive Care Unit? A Systematic Review and Meta-Analysis. *Shock*. 2017;47(3):288-295. doi:10.1097/SHK.0000000000000769
227) Anna S, Aleksandra S, Piotr W, Gabriel N, Maria R, Micha S, Ewa P. Magnesium in depression. Pharmacol Rep. 2013;65(3):547-54.
228) George A.Eby, Karen L. Eby Rapid recovery from major depression using magnesium treatment. Medical Hypotheses. 2006; 67, 2:362-370.

229) Emily K., Benjamin L, Charles D. M, Amanda G. K, Christopher D. Role of magnesium supplementation in the treatment of depression: A randomized clinical trial. Plos one; 2017.https://doi.org/10.1371/journal.pone.0180067
230) Eby GA, Eby KL. Rapid recovery from major depression using magnesium treatment. Med Hypotheses. 2006 67(2), 362-70.
231) Samad N, Yasmin F, Manzoor N. Biomarkers in Drug Free Subjects with Depression: Correlation with Tryptophan. Psychiatry Investig. 2019; 16(12):948-953. Published online November 13, 2019 DOI: https://doi.org/10.30773/pi.2019.0110
232) Ljungberg T, Bondza E, Lethin C. Evidence of the Importance of Dietary Habits Regarding Depressive Symptoms and Depression. Int J Environ Res Public Health. 2020; 2; 17(5):1616. doi: 10.3390/ijerph17051616. PMID: 32131552; PMCID: PMC7084175.
233) Boyle NB, Lawton C, Dye L. The Effects of Magnesium Supplementation on Subjective Anxiety and Stress-A Systematic Review. Nutrients. 2017; 26; 9(5):429. doi: 10.3390/nu9050429. PMID: 28445426; PMCID: PMC5452159.
234) Hemamy M, Heidari-Beni M, Askari G, Karahmadi M, Maracy M. Effect of Vitamin D and Magnesium Supplementation on Behavior Problems in Children with Attention-Deficit Hyperactivity Disorder. Int J Prev Med. 2020; 24; 11:4. doi: 10.4103/ijpvm.IJPVM_546_17. PMID: 32089804; PMCID: PMC7011463.
235) Starobat-Hermelin B, Kozielec T. The effects of magnesium physiological supplementation on hyperactive disorder (ADHD). Magnes Res. 1997; 10: 149-156.
236) Nechifor M. Interactions between magnesium and psychotropic drugs. Magnes Res. 2008; 21(2): 97-100.
237) Andrew W, Kristen N G, Tyler B G, and Vicki L. Ellingrod Schizophrenia and folate pharmacogenetics: Review of the literature regarding folic acid and its pharmacogenetically regulated metabolism in relation to schizophrenia treatments. Mental Health Clinician. 2012;1, 9, :225-229.
238) Fairbanks VF, Klee GG: Biochemical aspects of hematology. In Tietz Textbook of Clinical Chemistry. Edited by CA Burtis, ER Ashwood. Philadelphia, WB Saunders Company. 1999; 1690-1698
239) George L, Mills JL, Johansson AL, Anna N, Bodil O, Fredrik G, Sven C.Plasma folate levels and risk of spontaneous abortion. JAMA 2002; 288:1867-1873
240) Institute of Medicine (US) Standing Committee on the Scientific Evaluation of Dietary Reference Intakes and its Panel on Folate, Other B Vitamins, and Choline.
241) Zhao Y, Guo C, Hu H, Zheng L, Ma J, Jiang L, Zhao E, Li H. Folate intake, serum folate levels and esophageal cancer risk: an overall and dose-response

meta-analysis. Oncotarget. 2017; 7; 8 (6):10458-10469. doi: 10.18632/oncotarget.14432. PMID: 28060731; PMCID: PMC5354672.
242) Saedisomeolia A, Djalali M, Moghadam AM, Ramezankhani O, Najmi L. Folate and vitamin B12 status in schizophrenic patients. J Res Med Sci. 2011; 16 Suppl 1(Suppl1):S437-41. PMID: 22247731; PMCID: PMC3252772.
243) Roffman JL, Brohawn DG, Nitenson AZ, Macklin EA, Smolle JW, Goff DC, Genetic Variation Throughout the Folate Metabolic Pathway Influences Negative Symptom Severity in Schizophrenia, Schizophrenia Bulletin, 2013; 39, (2),:330–338, https://doi.org/10.1093/schbul/sbr150
244) Friso S, Choi SW. Gene-nutrient interactions in one-carbon metabolism. Curr Drug Metab. 2005; 6(1):37–46. PubMed PMID: 15720206.
245) Yamada K, Chen Z, Rozen R, Matthews RG. Effects of common polymorphisms on the properties of recombinant human methylenetetrahydrofolate reductase. Proc Natl Acad Sci U S A. 2001; 18; 98(26):14853-8. doi: 10.1073/pnas.261469998. Epub 2001 Dec 11. PMID:
246) Siew C, Geok K and Su-P L. Association between Dietary Folate Intake and Blood Status of Folate and Homocysteine in Malaysian Adults. J Nutr Sci Vitaminol. 2011; 57, 150–155.
247) Geok L K, Duraisamy G, Su P L, Timothy J G and Murray C S. Original Article Dietary and blood folate status of Malaysian women of childbearing age Asia Pac J Clin Nutr 2006;15 (3): 341-349341.
248) Bailey LB, Rampersaud GC, Kauwell GP. Folic acid supplements and fortification affect the risk for neural tube defects, vascular disease and cancer: evolving science. J Nutr. 2003; 133:1961S–1968S
249) Gerald Martone. Enhancement of recovery from mental illness with l-methylfolate supplementation. Perspectives in psychiatric practice. 2018; vol 24 (2)331-334
250) Owen RT. Augmenting antidepressant response with folates. Drugs Today. 2013; 49(12):791-8. doi: 10.1358/dot.2013.49.12.2086138
251) Coppen, A., & Bolander-Gouaille, C. Treatment of depression: time to consider folic acid and vitamin B12. Journal of Psychopharmacology. 2005; 19(1), 59–65. https://doi.org/10.1177
252) Roffman JL, Petruzzi LJ, Tanner AS, Brown HE, Eryilmaz H, Ho NF, Giegold M, Silverstein NJ, Bottiglieri T, Manoach DS, Smoller JW, Henderson DC, Goff DC. Biochemical, physiological and clinical effects of l-methylfolate in schizophrenia: a randomized controlled trial. Mol Psychiatry. 2018; 23(2):316-322. doi: 10.1038/mp.2017.41. Epub 2017 Mar 14. PMID: 28289280; PMCID: PMC5599314
253) Menegas S, Dal-Pont GC, Cararo JH, Roger V, Jorge M, Taise P, Monica A, Quevedo J, Samira V. Efficacy of folic acid as an adjunct to lithium therapy on manic-like behaviors, oxidative stress and inflammatory parameters in

an animal model of mania. Metab Brain Dis.2020; **35,** 413–42. https://doi.org/10.1007

254) Ma F, Wu T, Zhao J, Song A, Liu H, Xu W, Huang G. Folic acid supplementation improves cognitive function by reducing the levels of peripheral inflammatory cytokines in elderly Chinese subjects with MCI. Sci Rep. 2016; 23; 6: 37486. doi: 10.1038/srep37486. PMID: 27876835; PMCID: PMC5120319.

255) Petrilli MA, Kranz TM, Kleinhaus K, Joe P, Getz M, Johnson P, Chao MV, Malaspina D. The Emerging Role for Zinc in Depression and Psychosis. Front Pharmacol. 2017; 30; 8:414. doi: 10.3389/fphar.2017.00414. PMID: 28713269; PMCID: PMC5492454.

256) Takeda A. Zinc homeostasis and functions of zinc in the brain. Biometals. 2001; 14:343–351.

257) Smart TG, Hosie AM, Miller PS. Zn^{2+} ions: modulators of excitatory and inhibitory synaptic activity. Neuroscientist. 2004; 10: 432–442

258) Prasad A S Zinc: an overview. Nutrition. ; 1995: 11(1 Suppl), 93–99.

259) Marger L, Schubert CR, Bertrand D Zinc: an underappreciated modulatory factor of brain function. Biochem Pharmacol. 2014; 91(4):426-35.

260) Hess S Y, Peerson, J M, King J C, & Brown K. Use of Serum Zinc Concentration as an Indicator of Population Zinc Status. Food and Nutrition Bulletin. 2007: 28(3_suppl3), S403–S429.

261) Kumssa DB, Joy EJ, Ander EL, Watts MJ, Young SD, Walker S, Broadley MR. Dietary calcium and zinc deficiency risks are decreasing but remain prevalent. Sci Rep. 2015;22;5:10974. doi: 10.1038/srep10974. PMID: 26098577; PMCID: PMC4476434.

262) Kumar V, Sinha A K, Makkar H P S. & Becker K. Dietary roles of phytate and phytase in human nutrition: A review. Food Chem. 2010; 120, 945–959.

263) Norhaizan M. & Ain Nor Faizadatul A. Determination of phytate, iron, zinc, calcium contents and their molar ratios in commonly consumed raw and prepared food in Malaysia. Malays. J. Nutr.2009; 15, 213–222.

264) Nowak G. Does interaction between zinc and glutamate system play a significant role in the mechanism of antidepressant action? Acta Pol.2001; Pharm. 8, 73–75.

265) McLoughlin I J, Hodge J S. Zinc in depressive disorder. Acta Psychiatr. Scand.1990; 82, 451–453. 10.1111/j.1600-0447.1990.tb03077.x

266) Maes M, D'Haese P C, Scharpé S, D'Hondt P, Cosyns P, De Broe M E. Hypozincemia in depression. J. Affect. Disord. 1994; 31, 135–140. 10.1016/0165-0327(94)90117-1

267) Siwek M, Dudek D, Schlegel-Zawadzka M, Morawska A, Piekoszewski W, Opoka W, et al. Serum zinc level in depressed patients during zinc supplementation of imipramine treatment. J. Affect. Disord.2010; 126, 447–452. 10.1016/j.jad.2010.04.024

268) Swardfager W, Herrmann N, Mazereeuw G, Goldberger K, Harimoto T, Lanctôt K L. Zinc in depression: a meta-analysis. Biol. Psychiatry. 2013; 74, 872–878. 10.1016/j.biopsych.2013.05.008
269) Grabrucker A M, Rowan M, Garner C C. Brain-delivery of zinc-ions as potential treatment for neurological diseases: mini review. Drug Deliv. Lett.2013; 1, 13–23. 10.2174/2210304x11101010013
270) Liuzzi J P, Cousins R J. Mammalian zinc transporters. Annu Rev. Nutr.2014; 24, 151–172. 10.1146/annurev.nutr.24.012003.132402
271) Ranjbar E, Shams J, Sabetkasaei M, Shirazi M, Rashidkhani B, Mostafavi A, et al. Effects of zinc supplementation on efficacy of antidepressant therapy, inflammatory cytokines, and brain-derived neurotrophic factor in patients with major depression. Nutr. Neurosci.2014; 17, 65–71. 10.1179/1476830513Y.0000000066
272) Solati Z, Jazayeri S, Tehrani-Doost M, Mahmoodianfard S, Gohari MR Zinc monotherapy increases serum brain-derived neurotrophic factor (BDNF) levels and decreases depressive symptoms in overweight or obese subjects: a double-blind, randomized, placebo-controlled trial. Nutr Neurosci. 2015; 18(4):162-8.
273) Lai J., Moxey A., Nowak G., Vashum K., Bailey K., McEvoy M. (2012). The efficacy of zinc supplementation in depression: systematic review of randomised controlled trials. J. Affect. Disord. 136, e31–e39. 10.1016/j.jad.2011.06.022
274) Sawada T, Yokoi K. Effect of zinc supplementation on mood states in young women: a pilot study. Eur. J. Clin. Nutr.2010; 64, 331–333. 10.1038/ejcn.2009.158
275) Doboszewska U, Sowa-Kućma M, Młyniec K, et al. Zinc deficiency in rats is associated with up-regulation of hippocampal NMDA receptor. Prog Neuropsychopharmacol Biol Psychiatry. 201; 56:254-263.
276) Maserejian NN, Hall SA, McKinlay JB: Low dietary or supplemental zinc is associated with depression symptoms among women, but not men, in a population-based epidemiological survey. J Affect Disord 2012; 136:781–788.
277) Szewczyk B, Pochwat B, Rafało A, Palucha-Poniewiera A, Domin H, Nowak G. Activation of mTOR dependent signaling pathway is a necessary mechanism of antidepressant-like activity of zinc. Neuropharmacology. 2015; 99:517-26.
278) Xu H, Gao HL, Zheng W, Xin N, Chi ZH, Bai SL, Wang ZY. Lactational zinc deficiency-induced hippocampal neuronal apoptosis by a BDNF-independent TrkB signaling pathway. Hippocampus. 2011 May; 21(5):495-501.
279) Frazzini V, Granzotto A, Bomba M, Massetti N, Castelli V, d'Aurora M, Punzi M, Iorio M, Mosca A, Delli Pizzi S, Gatta V, Cimini A, Sensi SL. The pharmacological perturbation of brain zinc impairs BDNF-related signaling and the cognitive performances of young mice. Sci Rep. 2018; 27; 8(1):9768. doi: 10.1038/s41598-018-28083-9. PMID: 29950603; PMCID: PMC6021411.

280) Huang Y Z, Pan E, Xiong Z Q, McNamara J O. Zinc-mediated transactivation of TrkB potentiates the hippocampal mossy fiber-CA3 pyramid synapse. Neuron. 2008; 57, 546–558. 10.1016/j.neuron.2007.11.026
281) Pan E. Vesicular zinc promotes presynaptic and inhibits postsynaptic long-term potentiation of mossy fiber-CA3 synapse. Neuron. 2011; 71, 1116–1126. 10.1016/j.neuron.2011.07.019
282) Szewczyk B, Kata R, Nowak G. Rise in zinc affinity for the NMDA receptor evoked by chronic imipramine is species-specific. Pol J Pharmacol. 2001; 53(6):641-645.
283) Maes M, Vandoolaeghe E, Neels H, et al. Lower serum zinc in major depression is a sensitive marker of treatment resistance and of the immune/inflammatory response in that illness. Biol Psychiatry. 1997; 42(5):349-358. doi :10.1016/S0006-3223(96)00365-4.
284) Ilouz R, Kaidanovich O, Gurwitz D, and Eldar-Finkelman H, "Inhibition of glycogen synthase kinase-3β by bivalent zinc ions: insight into the insulin-mimetic action of zinc," Biochemical and Biophysical Research Communications 2002; 295, 1:102–106.
285) Meijer L, Flajolet M, Greengard P. Pharmacological inhibitors of glycogen synthase kinase 3. Trends in pharmacological sciences. 2004 Sep 1; 25(9):471-80.
286) Joe P, Petrilli M, Malaspina D, Weissman J. Zinc in schizophrenia: A meta-analysis. Gen Hosp Psychiatry. 2018; 53:19-24. doi:10.1016/j.genhosppsych.2018.04.004
287) Saghazadeh A, Mahmoudi M, Shahrokhi S, et al. Trace elements in schizophrenia: a systematic review and meta-analysis of 39 studies (N = 5151 participants). Nutr Rev. 2020;78(4):278-303. doi:10.1093/nutrit/nuz059.
288) Liu T, Lu QB, Yan L, et al. Comparative Study on Serum Levels of 10 Trace Elements in Schizophrenia. PLoS One. 2015; 10(7):e0133622. doi:10.1371/journal.pone.0133622.
289) Yanik M, Kocyigit A, Tutkun H, Vural H, Herken H. Plasma manganese, selenium, zinc, copper, and iron concentrations in patients with schizophrenia. Biol Trace Elem Res. 2004; 98(2):109-117. doi :10.1385/BTER:98:2:109.
290) Olatunbosun DA, Akindele MO, Adadevoh BK, Asuni T. Serum copper in schizophrenia in Nigerians. Br J Psychiatry. 1975; 127:119-121. doi:10.1192/bjp.127.2.119.
291) Arinola G, Idonije B, Akinlade K, Ihenyen O. Essential trace metals and heavy metals in newly diagnosed schizophrenic patients and those on anti-psychotic medication. J Res Med Sci. 2010 Sep; 15(5):245-9. PMID: 21526091; PMCID: PMC3082825.
292) Torres-Vega A, Pliego-Rivero BF, Otero-Ojeda GA, Gómez-Oliván LM, Vieyra-Reyes P. Limbic system pathologies associated with deficiencies and

excesses of the trace elements iron, zinc, copper, and selenium. Nutr Rev. 2012; 70(12):679-692. doi:10.1111/j.1753-4887.2012.00521.x

293) Mortazavi M, Farzin D, Zarhghami M, Hosseini SH, Mansoori P, Nateghi G. Efficacy of Zinc Sulfate as an Add-on Therapy to Risperidone Versus Risperidone Alone in Patients With Schizophrenia: A Double-Blind Randomized Placebo-Controlled Trial. Iran J Psychiatry Behav Sci. 2015 Sep;9(3):e853. doi: 10.17795/ijpbs-853. Epub 2015 Sep 23. PMID: 26576178; PMCID: PMC4644625.

294) Derek E, Joshua B, Askren M, Marc B, Emre D, Adam K and Jonides, J. 2015. A Meta-analysis of Executive Components of Working Memory. Cerebral Cortex, 23 (2), 264-282.

295) Vyas, J.V and Shree, R. 2015. Essentials of Postgraduate Psychiatry. 2 nd ed: Paras Publisher, pg 145.

296) Randi, C.M. and Robert, S. 2014.Language Production and Working Memory. The Oxforfd Handbook of Language Production. 1st ed Oxford. Oxford Press.

297) Bandura A. 1986 Social Foundations of Thought and Action: A Social Cognitive Theory. Englewood Cliffs, N.J.: Prentice-Hall.

298) Dudai, Y. 2002. Memory from A to Z: Keywords, concepts, and beyond. 1st ed Oxford, UK: Oxford University Press.

299) Purves D, Augustine GJ, Fitzpatrick D, Hall WC, Lamantia AS, McNamara JO, White LE. Neuroscience. 2008. 4th ed. Sunderland, MA. Sinauer Associates.

300) Adams F. The genuine works of Hippocrates: W. Wood; 1886.

301) Organization WH. Depression and other common mental disorders: global health estimates. World Health Organization; 2017.

302) Sullivan PF, Neale MC, Kendler KS. Genetic epidemiology of major depression: review and meta-analysis. American Journal of Psychiatry. 2000; 157(10):1552-62.

303) Cai N, Bigdeli TB, Kretzschmar W, Li Y, Liang J, Song L, et al. Sparse whole-genome sequencing identifies two loci for major depressive disorder. Nature. 2015;523(7562):588-91.

304) Howard DM, Adams MJ, Clarke T-K, Hafferty JD, Gibson J, Shirali M, et al. Genome-wide meta-analysis of depression in 807,553 individuals identifies 102 independent variants with replication in a further 1,507,153 individuals. bioRxiv. 2018:433367.

305) Heim C, Binder EB. Current research trends in early life stress and depression: Review of human studies on sensitive periods, gene–environment interactions, and epigenetics. Experimental neurology. 2012; 233(1):102-11.

306) Peyrot WJ, Middeldorp CM, Jansen R, Smit JH, de Geus EJ, Hottenga J-J, et al. Strong effects of environmental factors on prevalence and course of major

depressive disorder are not moderated by 5-HTTLPR polymorphisms in a large Dutch sample. Journal of affective disorders. 2013;146(1):91-9.

307) Llorente JM, Oliván-Blázquez B, Zuñiga-Antón M, Masluk B, Andrés E, García-Campayo J, et al. Variability of the prevalence of depression in function of sociodemographic and environmental factors: Ecological model. Frontiers in psychology. 2018;9:2182.

308) Wankerl M, Miller R, Kirschbaum C, Hennig J, Stalder T, Alexander N. Effects of genetic and early environmental risk factors for depression on serotonin transporter expression and methylation profiles. Translational psychiatry. 2014;4(6):e402-e.

309) Sjöberg RL, Nilsson KW, Nordquist N, Öhrvik J, Leppert J, Lindström L, et al. Development of depression: sex and the interaction between environment and a promoter polymorphism of the serotonin transporter gene. International Journal of Neuropsychopharmacology. 2006;9(4):443-9.

310) Piechaczek CE, Greimel E, Feldmann L, Pehl V, Allgaier A-K, Frey M, et al. Interactions between FKBP5 variation and environmental stressors in adolescent Major Depression. Psychoneuroendocrinology. 2019;106:28-37.

311) Power M. Mood disorders: A handbook of science and practice: John Wiley & Sons; 2004.

312) Ferrari F, Villa R. The neurobiology of depression: an integrated overview from biological theories to clinical evidence. Molecular neurobiology. 2017;54(7):4847-65.

313) Nemeroff CB, Vale WW. The neurobiology of depression: inroads to treatment and new drug discovery. The Journal of clinical psychiatry. 2005;66:5-13.

314) Carroll B, Cassidy F, Naftolowitz D, Tatham N, Wilson W, Iranmanesh A, et al. Pathophysiology of hypercortisolism in depression. Acta Psychiatrica Scandinavica. 2007;115:90-103.

315) Dowlati Y, Herrmann N, Swardfager WL, Reim EK, Lanctot KL. Efficacy and tolerability of antidepressants for treatment of depression in coronary artery disease: a meta-analysis. The Canadian Journal of Psychiatry. 2010;55(2):91-9.

316) Iwata M, Ota KT, Duman RS. The inflammasome: pathways linking psychological stress, depression, and systemic illnesses. Brain, behavior, and immunity. 2013;31:105-14.

317) Irwin MR, Miller AH. Depressive disorders and immunity: 20 years of progress and discovery. Brain, behavior, and immunity. 2007;21(4):374-83.

318) Association AP. Diagnostic and statistical manual of mental disorders (DSM-5®): American Psychiatric Pub; 2013.

319) Angst J, Sellaro R. Historical perspectives and natural history of bipolar disorder. Vol. 48, Biological Psychiatry. Elsevier; 2000. p. 445–57.

320) Wong NCH, Lookadoo KL, Nisbett GS. "I'm Demi and I Have Bipolar Disorder": Effect of Parasocial Contact on Reducing Stigma Toward People

With Bipolar Disorder. Commun Stud [Internet]. 2017 May 27 [cited 2020 Apr 2];68(3):314–33. Available from: https://www.tandfonline.com/doi/full/10.1080/10510974.2017.1331928

321) Rowland TA, Marwaha S. Epidemiology and risk factors for bipolar disorder. Ther Adv Psychopharmacol. 2018 Sep;8(9):251–69.

322) Kroon JS, Wohlfarth TD, Dieleman J, Sutterland AL, Storosum JG, Denys D, et al. Incidence rates and risk factors of bipolar disorder in the general population: a population-based cohort study. Bipolar Disord [Internet]. 2013 May 1 [cited 2020 Apr 2];15(3):306–13. Available from: http://doi.wiley.com/10.1111/bdi.12058

323) Craddock N, Sklar P. Bipolar Disorder 1 - Genetics of bipolar disorder. Vol. 381, The Lancet. Lancet Publishing Group; 2013. p. 1654–62.

324) Barnett JH, Smoller JW. The genetics of bipolar disorder. Vol. 164, Neuroscience. Pergamon; 2009. p. 331–43.

325) McGuffin P, Rijsdijk F, Andrew M, Sham P, Katz R, Cardno A. The heritability of bipolar affective disorder and the genetic relationship to unipolar depression. Arch Gen Psychiatry. 2003 May 1;60(5):497–502.

326) Seifuddin F, Mahon PB, Judy J, Pirooznia M, Jancic D, Taylor J, et al. Meta-analysis of genetic association studies on bipolar disorder. Am J Med Genet Part B Neuropsychiatr Genet [Internet]. 2012 Jul 1 [cited 2020 Apr 6];159B(5):508–18. Available from: http://doi.wiley.com/10.1002/ajmg.b.32057

327) Gordovez FJA, McMahon FJ. The genetics of bipolar disorder. Vol. 25, Molecular Psychiatry. Springer Nature; 2020. p. 544–59.

328) Alloy LB, Abramson LY, Urosevic S, Walshaw PD, Nusslock R, Neeren AM. The psychosocial context of bipolar disorder: Environmental, cognitive, and developmental risk factors. Clin Psychol Rev. 2005 Dec 1;25(8):1043–75.

329) Post RM. The status of the sensitization/kindling hypothesis of bipolar disorder. Curr Psychos Ther Rep. 2004 Dec;2(4):135–41.

330) Talati A, Bao Y, Kaufman J, Shen L, Schaefer CA, Brown AS. Maternal Smoking During Pregnancy and Bipolar Disorder in Offspring. Am J Psychiatry [Internet]. 2013 Oct 1 [cited 2020 Apr 6];170(10):1178–85. Available from: http://ajp.psychiatryonline.org/doi/10.1176/appi.ajp.2013.12121500

331) Lee HC, Tsai SY, Lin HC. Seasonal variations in bipolar disorder admissions and the association with climate: A population-based study. J Affect Disord. 2007 Jan 1;97(1–3):61–9.

332) Aas M, Henry C, Andreassen OA, Bellivier F, Melle I, Etain B. The role of childhood trauma in bipolar disorders. Vol. 4, International Journal of Bipolar Disorders. SpringerOpen; 2016. p. 1–10.

333) Melo MCA, Abreu RLC, Linhares Neto VB, de Bruin PFC, de Bruin VMS. Chronotype and circadian rhythm in bipolar disorder: A systematic review. Vol. 34, Sleep Medicine Reviews. W.B. Saunders Ltd; 2017. p. 46–58.

334) Morris G, Walder K, McGee SL, Dean OM, Tye SJ, Maes M, et al. A model of the mitochondrial basis of bipolar disorder. Vol. 74, Neuroscience and Biobehavioral Reviews. Elsevier Ltd; 2017. p. 1–20.

335) Rowland T, Perry BI, Upthegrove R, Barnes N, Chatterjee J, Gallacher D, et al. Neurotrophins, cytokines, oxidative stress mediators and mood state in bipolar disorder: Systematic review and meta-analyses. Vol. 213, British Journal of Psychiatry. Cambridge University Press; 2018. p. 514–25.

336) Rosa AR, Singh N, Whitaker E, De Brito M, Lewis AM, Vieta E, et al. Altered plasma glutathione levels in bipolar disorder indicates higher oxidative stress; A possible risk factor for illness onset despite normal brain-derived neurotrophic factor (BDNF) levels. Psychol Med. 2014;44(11):2409–18.

337) Kim Y, Santos R, Gage FH, Marchetto MC. Molecular mechanisms of bipolar disorder: Progress made and future challenges. Vol. 11, Frontiers in Cellular Neuroscience. Frontiers Research Foundation; 2017. p. 30.

338) Chr Kyziridis T. Notes on the History of Schizophrenia. Ger J Psychiatry ·

339) Bark N. On the history of schizophrenia. Evidence of its existence before 1800 [Internet].

340) Fusar-Poli P, Politi P. Paul Eugen Bleuler and the Birth of Schizophrenia (1908). Am J Psychiatry [Internet]. 2008 Nov 1;165(11):1407–1407.

341) Schizophrenia in adults: Epidemiology and pathogenesis - UpToDate [Internet].

342) Getinet Ayano. Schizophrenia: A Concise Overview of Etiology, Epidemiology Diagnosis and Management: Review of literatures [Internet]. 2016

343) Schwartz RC. Racial disparities in psychotic disorder diagnosis: A review of empirical literature. World J Psychiatry. 2014;4(4):133.

344) Cardno AG, Gottesman II. Twin studies of schizophrenia: From bow-and-arrow concordances to Star Wars Mx and functional genomics. Am J Med Genet. 2000 Mar 1;97(1):12–7.

345) Mulle JG. Schizophrenia genetics: Progress, at last. Vol. 22, Current Opinion in Genetics and Development. Elsevier Current Trends; 2012. p. 238–44.

346) Bergen SE, Petryshen TL. Genome-wide association studies of schizophrenia: Does bigger lead to better results? Vol. 25, Current Opinion in Psychiatry. NIH Public Access; 2012. p. 76–82.

347) Cannon M, Jones PB, Murray RM. Obstetric complications and schizophrenia: Historical and meta-analytic review. Vol. 159, American Journal of Psychiatry. American Psychiatric Publishing; 2002. p. 1080–92.

348) Clarke Mary, Kelleher Eoin. Obstetric Complications and Schizophrenia—Systematic Review and Meta-Analysis Update. Schizophr Bull [Internet]. 2017 Mar;43(1).

349) Lederbogen F, Haddad L, Meyer-Lindenberg A. Urban social stress—risk factor for mental disorders. The case of schizophrenia. Environ Pollut. 2013 Dec 1;183:2–6.

350) DeVylder JE, Kelleher I, Lalane M, Oh H, Link BG, Koyanagi A. Association of urbanicity with psychosis in low- and middle-income countries. JAMA Psychiatry. 2018 Jul 1;75(7):678–86.
351) Read J, Os J, Morrison AP, Ross CA. Childhood trauma, psychosis and schizophrenia: a literature review with theoretical and clinical implications. Acta Psychiatr Scand [Internet]. 2005 Nov 1;112(5):330–50.
352) Morgan Craig, Fisher Helen. Environment and Schizophrenia: Environmental Factors in Schizophrenia: Childhood Trauma—A Critical Review. Schizophr Bull [Internet]. 2007 Nov 1;33(1):3–10.
353) Vaucher J, Keating BJ, Lasserre AM, Gan W, Lyall DM, Ward J, et al. Cannabis use and risk of schizophrenia: A Mendelian randomization study. Mol Psychiatry. 2018 May 1;23(5):1287–92.
354) Verweij KJH, Abdellaoui A, Nivard MG, Sainz Cort A, Ligthart L, Draisma HHM, et al. Short communication: Genetic association between schizophrenia and cannabis use. Drug Alcohol Depend. 2017 Feb 1;171:117–21.
355) Voce A, McKetin R, Burns R, Castle D, Calabria B. The relationship between illicit amphetamine use and psychiatric symptom profiles in schizophrenia and affective psychoses. Psychiatry Res. 2018 Jul 1;265:19–24.
356) Fearon Paul, Morgan Craig. Environmental Factors in Schizophrenia: The Role of Migrant Studies. Schizophr Bull [Internet]. 2006 Jul ;32(3):405–8.
357) Karlsen S, Nazroo JY, McKenzie K, Bhui K, Weich S. Racism, psychosis and common mental disorder among ethnic minority groups in England. Psychol Med. 2005 Dec;35(12):1795–803.
358) Stone JM, Morrison PD, Pilowsky LS. Glutamate and dopamine dysregulation in schizophrenia - A synthesis and selective review [Internet]. Vol. 21, Journal of Psychopharmacology. 2007. p. 440–52.
359) Kuepper R, Skinbjerg M, Abi-Dargham A. The Dopamine Dysfunction in Schizophrenia Revisited: New Insights into Topography and Course. In Springer, Berlin, Heidelberg; 2012. p. 1–26.
360) Abi-Dargham A, Moore H. Prefrontal DA Transmission at D1 Receptors and the Pathology of Schizophrenia. Neurosci [Internet]. 2003 Oct 29;9(5):404–16. Available from: http://journals.sagepub.com/doi/10.1177/1073858403252674
361) Kirkpatrick Brian, Miller Brian J. Inflammation and Schizophrenia. Schizophr Bull [Internet]. 2013 Nov;39(6):1174–9.
362) Bitanihirwe BKY, Woo TUW. Oxidative stress in schizophrenia: An integrated approach.Vol. 35, Neuroscience and Biobehavioral Reviews. Pergamon; 2011. p. 878–93.
363) Gropper S, and Smith, J. Advanced Nutrition and Metabolism, 7th ed. Ohio: Cengage Learning; 2017.

364) Punia S, Sandhu K, Siroha A, Dhull S. Omega 3-metabolism, absorption, bioavailability and health benefits–A review. PharmaNutrition. 2019; 10:100162.
365) Lange K. Omega-3 fatty acids and mental health. Global Health Journal. 2020; doi: 10.1016/j.glohj.2020.01.004
366) Lerner P, Sharony L, Miodownik C. Association between mental disorders, cognitive disturbances and vitamin D serum level: Current state. Clinical Nutrition ESPEN. 2018; 23:89-102.
367) Norman AW, Henry HL. Vitamin D. In: Zempleni J, Rucker RB, McCormick DB, Suttie JW, editors. Handbook of vitamins. Boca Raton, Fl: CRC Press; 2007.p. 41e109.
368) Borel P, Caillaud D, Cano N. Vitamin D Bioavailability: State of the Art. Critical Reviews in Food Science and Nutrition. 2013; 55(9):1193-1205.
369) Partonen T. Vitamin D and serotonin in winter. Med Hypotheses 1998; 51:267e8.
370) Neumeister A, Konstantinidis A, Praschak-Rieder N, Willeit M, Hilger E, Stastny J, et al. Monoaminergic function in the pathogenesis of seasonal affectivedisorder. Int J Neuropsychopharmacol 2001; 4:409e20.
371) Stumpf WE, Privette TH. Light, vitamin D and psychiatry. Role of 1,25vdihydroxyvitamin D3 (soltriol) in etiology and therapy of seasonal affective disorder and other mental processes. Psychopharmacology 1989; 97: 285e94.
372) Maurya V, Aggarwal M. Factors influencing the absorption of vitamin D in GIT: an overview. Journal of Food Science and Technology. 2017; 54(12):3753-3765.
373) Compston JE, Merrett AL, Hammett F, Magill P. Comparison of the appearance of radiolabelled vitamin D3 and 25-hydroxy-vitamin D3 in the chylomicron fraction of plasma after oral administration in man. Clin Sci. 1981; 60: 241–243. doi: 10.1042/cs0600241.
374) Batchelor, A.J, and Compston, J.E. Reduced plasma half-life of radio-labelled 25- hydroxyvitamin D3 in subjects receiving a high-fibre diet. Br. J. Nutr. 1983; 49: 213-216.
375) Brügger B. Lipidomics: analysis of the lipid composition of cells and subcellular organelles by electrospray ionization mass spectrometry. Annu Rev Biochem. 2014; 83:79– 98.
376) Bowen KJ, Harris WS, Kris-Etherton PM. Omega-3 fatty acids and cardiovascular disease : are there benefits? Curr Treat Options Cardiovasc Med 2016; 18:69.
377) Fialkow J. Omega-3 fatty acid formulations in cardiovascular disease: dietary supplements are not substitutes for prescription products. Am J Cardiovasc Drugs 2016; 16:229– 239.

378) Balk EM, Lichtenstein AH. Omega-3 fatty acids and cardiovascular disease;summary of the 2016 Agency of Healthcare Research and Quality EvidenceReview. Nutrients 2017; 9: pii: E865.
379) Maki K, Dicklin M. Strategies to improve bioavailability of omega-3 fatty acids from ethyl ester concentrates. Current Opinion in Clinical Nutrition & Metabolic Care. 2019; 22(2):116-123.
380) Rudin DO. The major psychosis and neuroses as omega-3 essential fatty acid deficiency syndrome: substrate pellagra. Biol Psychiatry. 1981; 16(9):837–850.
381) Glen AL, Glen EM, Horrobin DF, Vaddadi KS, Spellman M, Morse F, Ellis K, Skinner F. A red cell membrane abnormality in a subgroup of schizophrenic patients: evidence for two diseases. Schizophr Res. 1994; 12(1):53–61.
382) Ross B, Seguin J, Sieswerda L. Omega-3 fatty acids as treatments for mental illness: which disorder and which fatty acid? Lipids in Health and Disease. 2007; 6(1):21.
383) Schuchardt JP, Schneider I, Meyer H, NeubronnerJ, von Schacky C, Hahn A. Incorporation of EPA and DHA into plasma phospholipids in response to different omega-3 fatty acid formulations-a comparative bioavailability study of fish oil vs. krill oil, Lipids Health Dis. 10 (1) (2011) 145, https://doi.org/10.1186/1476-511X- 10-145.
384) Ito MK. A comparative overview of prescription omega-3 fatty acid products. PT 2015; 40:826–857.
385) Fialkow J. Omega-3 fatty acid formulations in cardiovascular disease: dietary supplements are not substitutes for prescription products. Am J Cardiovasc Drugs 2016; 16:229–239.
386) Lawson LD, Hughes BG. Human absorption of fish oil fatty acids as triacylglycerols, free acids or ethyl esters. Biochem Biophys Res Commun 1998; 152:328–335.
387) Lawson LD, Hughes BG. Absorption of eicosapentaenoic acid and docosahexaenoicacid from docosa oil triacylglycerols or fish oil ethyl esters co-ingested with a high-fat meal. Biochem Biophys Res Commun 1988; 156:960–963.
388) Davidson MH, Johnson J, Rooney MW, Kyle M, Doughlas K. A novel omega-3 free fatty acid formulation has dramatically improved bioavailability during a low-fat diet compared with omega-3-acid ethyl esters: the ECLIPSE (Epanova (1) compared to Lovaza (1) in a pharmacokinetic single-dose evaluation) study. J ClinLipidol 2012; 6:573–584.
389) Offman E, Marenco T, Ferber S, Judith J, Douglas K, Danielle C, Michael D.Steady-state bioavailability of prescription omega-3 on a low-fat diet is significantly improved with a free fatty acid formulation compared with an ethyl ester formulation: the ECLIPSE II study. Vasc Health Risk Manag. 2013; 9:563–573.

www.ingramcontent.com/pod-product-compliance
Lightning Source LLC
Chambersburg PA
CBHW030805180526
45163CB00003B/1153